RENAL DIET COOKBOOK
FOR BEGINNERS

1500+ Days of Tasty Recipes For Every Stage of Kidney Disease. Low Sodium, Low Potassium and Low Phosphorus Meals. 35-Day Easy Meal Plan Included.

By Gina Ashley

Copyright © 2021 by Gina Ashley - All rights reserved.

This book may not be reproduced, duplicated or transmitted without direct written permission from the author or the publisher.

Legal Notice: This book is copyright protected. This book is only for personal use. You cannot amend, distribute, sell, use, quote or paraphrase any part of the content within this book without the written consent of the author or publisher.

Disclaimer Notice: This publication is designed to provide accurate and personal experience information in regard to the subject matter covered. It is sold with the understanding that the author, contributors, publisher are not engaged in rendering counseling or other professional services. If counseling advice or other expert assistance is required, the services of a competent professional person should be sought out.

No warranties of any kind are declared or implied. Readers acknowledge that the author is not engaging in the rendering of legal, financial, medical or professional advice.

The information contained in this book is not intended to serve as a replacement for professional medical advice. Any use of the information in this book is at the reader's discretion. The author and publisher specifically disclaim any and all liability arising directly or indirectly from the use or application of any information contained in this book. A health care professional should be consulted regarding your specific situation.

Trademarks that are mentioned within this book are for clarifying purpose only. Trademarks are mentioned without written consent and can in no way be considered an endorsement from the trademark holder.

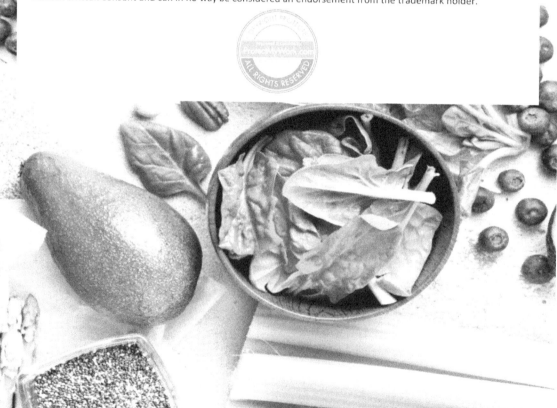

TABLE OF CONTENTS

Introduction _____ 7

Chapter 1. Kidney Disease Overview ___ 9
- How Kidneys Work _____ 9
- Chronic Kidney Disease from Stage 1 to 5 10

Chapter 2. Tips to Prevent Kidney Damage _____ 11
- Tips for Eating Salt _____ 12
- Tips Against Food Infections _____ 15

Chapter 3. Foods in Your Pantry _____ 16
- Foods to Eat and Foods to Avoid with Kidney Disease _____ 16
  - *Potassium* _____ 16
  - *Sodium* _____ 16
  - *Phosphorous* _____ 16
- Kidney-Friendly Dairy Alternatives _____ 17
- Kidney-Friendly Vegetables _____ 17
- Kidney-Friendly Fruits _____ 17
- Foods to be consumed in moderate quantities _____ 17
- Meat and Fish to be consumed in moderate quantities _____ 18
- Fats to be consumed in moderate quantities _____ 18

Chapter 4. Easy 5-Weeks Meal Plan ___ 19
- Week 1 plan _____ 19
- Week 2 Plan _____ 20
- Week 3 Plan _____ 21
- Week 4 Plan _____ 22
- Week 5 Plan _____ 23

Chapter 5. Breakfast _____ 24
- Bacon and Egg Tortilla _____ 24
- Cottage Cheese Pancakes _____ 24
- Egg in a Hole _____ 24
- German Pancakes _____ 25
- Mushroom and Red Pepper Omelet ____ 25
- Apple and Zucchini Bread _____ 25
- Spicy Corn Bread _____ 26
- Pumpkin Bread _____ 26
- Crunchy Potato Croquettes _____ 27
- Vegetarian Summer Rolls _____ 27
- Sour Cream and Apple Bread _____ 27
- Strawberry Bread _____ 28
- Zucchini Bread _____ 28
- Blistered Beans and Almond _____ 28
- Lemon and Broccoli Platter _____ 29
- Egg White and Pepper Omelet _____ 29
- Turkey Sausage _____ 29
- Italian Apple Fritters _____ 29
- Tofu and Mushroom Scramble _____ 30
- Egg Fried Rice _____ 30
- Lemon and Berry Bread _____ 30
- Asparagus Bacon Hash _____ 31
- Parmesan Zucchini Frittata _____ 31
- Mexican Baked Beans and Rice _____ 31
- Quick Thai Chicken and Vegetable Curry 32
- Cajun Stuffed Peppers _____ 32
- Stuffed Zucchinis _____ 33

Chapter 6. Soups _____ 34
- Chicken Fajita Soup _____ 34
- Italian Soup _____ 34

Cream of Chicken Soup	35
Green Chicken Enchilada Soup	35
Beef Stew	35
Bacon Cheeseburger Soup	36
Red Pepper & Brie Soup	36
Turkey & Lemon-Grass Soup	36
Paprika Pork Soup	37
Mediterranean Vegetable Soup	37
Tofu and Zucchini Soup	37
Onion Soup	38
Roasted Red Pepper Soup	38
Chicken Soup	38
Chicken and Rice Soup	39
Tomato and Bean Soup	39
Pan-Fried White Fish Soup	39
Vegetable Soup	39
Carrot and Ginger Soup	40
Cream of Mushroom Soup	40

Chapter 7. Sauces and Seasoning Mixes 41

Basil Pesto Sauce	41
Jalapeño Tomato Salsa	41
Seafood Seasoning	41
Pizza Sauce	41
Chicken and Turkey Seasoning	42
Garlicky Sauce	42
Pepper and Lemon Seasoning	42
Edamame Guacamole	42
Sweet Vinegar Sauce	43
BBQ Dry Rub	43
Cranberry Cabbage	43
Cajun Seasoning	43
White Alfredo Sauce	44
Vinaigrette	44
Healthy Mayonnaise	44
Tzatziki Sauce	44
Asian Seasoning	45
Creole Seasoning	45
Yogurt Cream Sauce	45
Broccoli and Garlic Sauce	45
Taco Sauce	46

Chapter 8. Snacks 47

Cereal Munch	47
Coconut Mandarin Salad	47
Cream Dipped Cucumbers	47
Puff Pastry Barbecue Cups	47
Spiced Pretzels	48
Seafood Croquettes	48
Falafel Balls	48
Spiced Tortilla Chips	49
Almond Caramel Corn	49
Sweet Popped Popcorn	49
Cranberry Pecan Salad	49
Carrot Corn Bread	50
Spiced Tortilla Chips	50
Tuna Dip	50
Chicken Bacon Wraps	50

Chapter 9. Salads 52

Pineapple Cabbage Coleslaw	52
Lemon peppers salad	52
Healthy Italian Pinzimonio	52
Sweet Rice Salad	52
Blue Cheese Pear Salad	53
Fresh salad	53

Chapter 10. Meat and Poultry Mains 54

Chicken in Herb Sauce	54
Chicken with Garlic Sauce	54

Chicken with Mushroom Sauce	54
Beef chorizo	55
Basil Lemon Turkey	55
Lamb with Prunes	55
Cabbage Rolls with Chicken	56
Turkey and Apple Curry	56
Beef and Three Pepper Stew	57
Sticky Pulled Beef Open Sandwiches	57
Herby Beef Stroganoff and Fluffy Rice	57
Chunky Beef and Potato Slow Roast	58
Chicken and Dumplings	58
Chicken Lasagna with White Sauce	58
Chicken with Cornbread Stuffing	59
Spiced Lamb Burgers	59
Chicken Stuffed Avocado	59
Pork Loins with Leeks	60
Chinese Beef Wraps	60
Grilled Skirt Steak	60
Spicy Lamb Curry	61
Sweet and Sour Chicken	61
Roast Beef	61
Beef Brochettes	62
Fajitas from Turkey	62
Country Fried Steak	62
Apple Spice Pork Chops	63
Crispy Sesame Chicken	63
Garlic Chicken with Balsamic Vinegar	63
Turkey Breast with Cranberry Gravy	64
Grilled Pineapple Chicken	64
Chicken Enchiladas	64

Chapter 11. Fish and Seafood Mains ___ 66

Shrimp Paella	66
Herbed Shrimps	66
Salmon & Pesto Salad	66
Garlic Flavored Cod	67
Baked Fennel & Garlic Sea Bass	67
Lemon, Garlic & Cilantro Tuna and Rice	67
Cod & Green Bean Risotto	67
Sardine Fish Cakes	68
Cajun Catfish	68
Sage Salmon Fillet	68
Spanish Cod in Sauce	69
Fish Shakshuka	69
Salmon Baked in Foil with Fresh Thyme	69
Poached Halibut in Lemon Sauce	70
Fish Papillote	70
Tuna Casserole	70
Oregano Salmon with Crunchy Crust	70
Ginger Shrimp with Snow Peas	71
Fish Chili with Lentils	71
Chili Mussels	71
Fried Scallops in Heavy Cream	72
Lettuce Seafood Wraps	72
Mango Tilapia Fillets	72
Roasted Cod with Plums	73
Family Hit Curry	73
Homemade Tuna Nicoise	73
Cajun Crab	74
Creamy Crab Soup	74
Spicy Lime Shrimp	74
Seafood Casserole	74
Tilapia Ceviche	75
Fish Tacos	75

Chapter 12. Vegetarian Mains ___ 76

Grilled Squash	76
Delicious Vegetarian Lasagna	76

Chili Tofu Noodles	76
Curried Cauliflower	77
Elegant Veggie Tortillas	77
Sweet and Sour Chickpeas	77
Cabbage-Stuffed Mushrooms	78
Curried Veggie Stir-Fry	78
Creamy Mushroom Pasta	78
Chinese Tempeh Stir Fry	79
Broccoli with Garlic Butter and Almonds	79
Eggplant French Fries	79
Thai Tofu Broth	80
Broccoli Steaks	80
Roasted Garlic Lemon Cauliflower	80
Veg Stew	81
Couscous with Vegetables	81
Grill Thyme Corn on the Cob	81
Ginger Glazed Carrots	82
Sautéed Green Beans	82
Carrot-Apple Casserole	82
Broccoli-Onion Latkes	82
Eggplant Casserole	83
Asparagus Quiche	83
Spinach Egg Bake	83
Vegetarian Quinoa Chili	84
Stuffed Bell Pepper	84
Zucchini Eggplant with Cheese	84

Chapter 13. Desserts _____ 85

Chocolate Beet Cake	85
Strawberry Pie	85
Pumpkin Cheesecake	86
Small Chocolate Cakes	86
Strawberry Whipped Cream Cake	86
Sweet Cracker Pie Crust	87
Apple Oatmeal Crunchy	87
Berry Ice Cream	87
Blueberry Peach Crisp	87
Cherry Coffee Cake	88
Fruity Peach Crisp Dump	88
Gingersnap Cookies	88
Lemon Icebox Pie	89
Strawberry Pavlova	89
Snickerdoodles	89
Bread Pudding	90
Frozen Fruit Delight	90
Italian Tiramisu Cheesecake	90
Frozen Lemon Dessert	91
Chocolate Pie Shell	91

Conclusion _____ 93

Introduction

Inside your body, two fist-sized organs sit below your rib cage and toward your back: your kidneys. Kidneys are your body's natural filtration system that helps eliminate excess water and waste from the body. When these organs become damaged over a long time and begin to decrease in function, this is called chronic kidney disease (CKD for short).

CKD does not have a sudden onset but instead happens slowly and over a long period. If this is not treated, it can cause excess water and waste to build up in your body. If this build-up occurs, many CKD patients use dialysis as a blood filtration because their kidneys can't handle the work. If dialysis is not an option or the disease has progressed too far for dialysis to work, a transplant may be necessary.

People living with type 1 or type 2 diabetes, or high blood pressure seem to have a higher risk of getting CKD in their lifetime. Research has also found that heart disease and a family history of kidney failure may significantly increase the chances of a person developing CKD. The opportunity of CKD also increases with age. Living with high blood pressure, heart disease, or diabetes for an extended time increases these risks.

There are over thirty million American adults living with CKD. Native Americans and those of African and Hispanic descent are more at risk than those who are not. These ethnicities have higher rates of diabetes and high blood pressure, making them vulnerable to the disease.

The following chart shows the adult population in the United States and the percentages for CKD, diabetes,

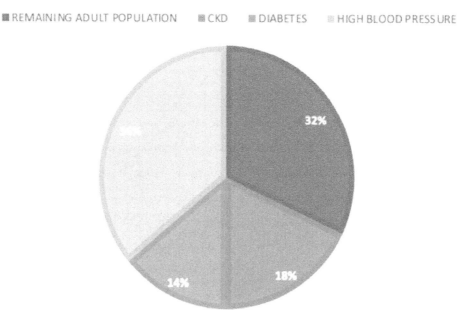

and high blood pressure.

Initially, CKD can develop slowly and silently, making it difficult to identify. As the illness worsens, symptoms include weariness, swelling, altered urination, cramping and twitching of the muscles, nausea and vomiting, itching, and dry skin may appear. Regular renal function testing is advised for people at risk, and early detection and treatment of CKD are crucial to preventing the build-up of toxins in the body. The first thing to do, and the most important if you are among the at-risk population or have any of the symptoms described above, is to see a doctor. Kidney disease is critical and needs health care from qualified physicians.

That said, once you have consulted your physician and established that you need a kidney-specific diet, this book can be a priceless tool to help you deal with the change in diet.

In the beginning, you will find an overview of the various stages of kidney disease and precious tips for lowering kidney-damaging nutrients. From appetizers to desserts and snacks, you will have a wide variety of tasty recipes that will make you forget you are on a diet.

Managing chronic kidney disease can be challenging, but with this cookbook, you can be sure you are in good hands. I have carefully crafted tasty and nutritious recipes designed to support kidney health. By incorporating these recipes into your diet, you can maintain healthy blood pressure and blood sugar levels while receiving the essential nutrients your body needs. In this book, you can get practical tips and advice on how to make dietary changes that can help prevent the progression of kidney disease.

Chapter 1. Kidney Disease Overview

The stage of kidney deterioration known as chronic kidney disease, or CKD, occurs when the kidneys cannot adequately filter blood. Chronic organ damage is characterized as being slow-moving and ongoing. Thus, chronic kidney disease develops due to gradual but irreversible kidney damage. Only when the body's toxic wastes begin to accumulate do the disease's symptoms begin to show. Therefore, it is imperative to avoid such a stage at all costs. Because of this, early disease diagnosis is crucial.

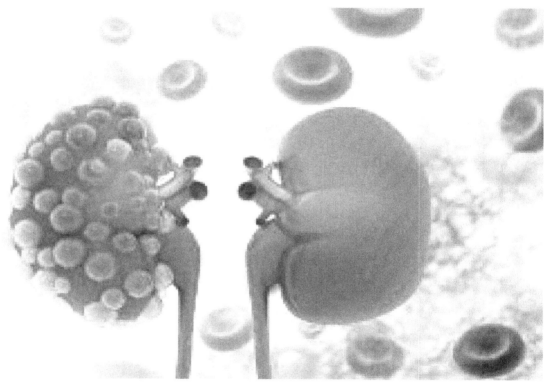

How Kidneys Work

Humans have two kidneys, one on the left and one on the right. Both kidneys perform important tasks in the body:

- Elimination of metabolic end products (so-called urinary substances: creatinine, urea, uric acid) and medications.
- Keeping the water balance constant.
- Regulation of the electrolyte balance.
- Maintaining the acid-base balance.
- Formation of hormones (such as erythropoietin and renin).
- Conversion of inactive to active vitamin D.
- Blood pressure regulation.

Chronic Kidney Disease from Stage 1 to 5

Chronic kidney disease failure is divided into five stages based on the glomerular filtration rate (GFR). The GFR shows how well the kidneys excrete urinary substances (especially creatinine and urea). Their normal value is 95 to 120 ml per minute / 1.73 square meters of the body surface. This means a healthy kidney removes at least 95 ml of blood from creatinine and other small-molecule poisonous substances per minute and excretes them with the urine.

Stage 1

GFR greater than 90 ml/min.

It is mostly a coincidence. The kidney detoxification function is still normal; the patient has no complaints from this side. The blood levels of the urinary substances are normal, but blood or **Protein:** may already be excreted in the urine. If this happens in large quantities, it can lead to symptoms.

Stage 2

GFR between 60 to 89 ml/min.

There are still no symptoms, but if the diagnosis is precise, there is a restriction of the detoxification function of the kidneys and the first other laboratory changes (parathyroid hormone increases).

Stage 3

GFR between 30 to 59 ml/min.

The kidney damage has progressed so much that increased creatinine and urea values usually also occur in the blood. Those affected complain of high blood pressure (hypertension), reduced performance, and rapid fatigue due to secondary complications such as anemia.

Stage 4

GFR between 15 to 29 ml/min.

Victims suffer from ailments such as loss of appetite, vomiting, nausea, nerve pain, itching, and bone pain or edema. So many filter particles are already defective that the deficient excretion of the urinary substances affects the entire organism. However, there is "not only" poisoning but also a lack of certain vital substances. Erythropoietin is no longer sufficiently produced in the kidney, which increases renal anemia (anemia). An overactive parathyroid gland interferes with vitamin D and bone metabolism.

Stage 5

GFR below 15 ml/min.

If the kidneys fail completely, one speaks of terminal renal failure. The organism must be cleaned of toxins by kidney replacement procedures.

Chapter 2. Tips to Prevent Kidney Damage

Maintaining a healthy lifestyle sounds so simple, but it is sometimes so difficult. Below you can read what a healthy lifestyle is and how to reduce the risk of kidney damage. Many of these recommendations will correspond to the lifestyle recommendations for high blood pressure and diabetes, diseases that can lead to kidney damage.

Healthy Food

Nutrition is most important when it comes to kidney disease at all stages. Eat varied, not too much, less saturated fat, less salt, lots of vegetables, lots of fruit, and enough bread.

Healthy Weight

People who are overweight have an increased risk of kidney damage (and other diseases such as diabetes and cardiovascular disease). It is, therefore, essential to strive for a healthy weight. The Body Mass Index (BMI) is used worldwide to determine whether someone has a healthy weight. So check regularly how your BMI is doing.

Enough Exercise

Modifying intensity for one hour of daily exercise is helpful for your health. That means you must breathe correctly, and your heart beats faster. Moving for half an hour does not have to be consecutive. Cycling twice for 15 minutes or walking ten times for 10 minutes is also possible.

Do Not Smoke

Smoking can damage the blood vessels in and towards the kidneys. It is, therefore, an important risk for kidney damage. Stopping smoking ensures that your health immediately jumps. And you notice it: your breathing improves, coughing becomes less, the condition increases, and smelling and tasting go better.

Moderate Drinking

For adult men and women, moderate drinking means, on average, no more than a standard glass per day. The benefits of drinking alcohol do not outweigh the disadvantages. That is why the advice is not to drink alcohol or at least not more than one glass per day. In any case, try to insert many alcohol-free days.

Regular check-ups

It is crucial to stay on top of your kidney health by scheduling regular check-ups with a healthcare provider. This way, any issues can be identified early on, and measures can be taken to prioritize preventative care.

Tips for Eating Salt

Eating less salt can delay the worsening of kidney damage. But it can be challenging to reduce salt. When you buy, much of the salt you get is already in the products. And you may have to get used to the taste of eating less salt.

These tips help you eat less salt:
- Give yourself time to get used to it.
- Choose unprocessed foods.
- Do not add salt yourself.
- Avoid salty seasonings.
- Use herbs, spices, and condiments such as onion and garlic.
- Eat less salty bread meals.
- Let someone else cook (sometimes).
- Avoid licorice, licorice tea, minty Maroc tea, and star mix tea.

Give Yourself Time to Get Used to It

Remember that it takes time to get used to a meal without salt. You have to get rid of the salty taste. This is only possible by consistently not using salt or salty seasonings. In the beginning, less salt food tastes mostly bland, but after a while, you will taste better and find a lot of salt dirty.

Choose Unprocessed Food

Processed foods are products that the manufacturer has processed with salt or other flavorings. These products contain (a lot of) salt. Think of ready-made sauces and soups and ready-made meals. Avoid processed meat, such as hamburgers, roulade, seasoned minced meat, and sausage. Also, do away with processed fish, such as marinated fresh fish, breaded (frozen) fish, steamed and smoked fish, and canned and pickled fish.

Therefore, choose unprocessed food: unprocessed meat, unprocessed chicken, unprocessed fish, and fresh vegetables or frozen vegetables. Season with herbs and spices if necessary.

Ask a butcher to prepare processed meat without salt, such as a low-sodium variant of processed meat like a roulade.

Choose vegetable preserves without added salt: look at the health food store or the supermarket diet.

Cook extra portions and store them in the freezer as an alternative to a salty ready-made meal.

Compare labels

Compare different brands and variants of food. The differences in the amount of salt are significant. Your salt intake will decrease if you always choose the brand or variant with the least salt.

Do Not Add Salt Yourself

Do not add any more salt by yourself when cooking. Place the salt pot far away so you do not grab it automatically.

Also, do not use salt products with other names. Such as:

Celery salt, garlic salt, onion salt, Himalayan salt, or Celtic sea salt. These contain just as much salt as common kitchen salt.

Dietary salt, half-salt, and mineral salt contain much less sodium than ordinary salt. Potassium is in it instead. If you have a potassium limitation, there are more suitable alternatives to salt than these products.

Monosodium glutamate (E621)

This flavor enhancer contains sodium. It is also known as Chinese salt or Ve-tsin.

Avoid Salty Seasonings

Avoid using salty seasonings—for example, Maggi, bouillon cubes, soy sauce, scattering aroma, and soy sauce.

Sodium-Limited Variant

A Sodium-limited version of many flavorings is also available. Ask about it at supermarkets or health food stores. Sodium-limited flavorings often contain potassium. Look at the label. Potassium is also listed as potassium chloride or E508. If you have potassium restriction, these sodium-restricted flavorings are not a suitable alternative.

Use Herbs- with herb seasoning recipe

Use fresh or dried garden herbs and spices to add flavor to your food.

Avoid ready-to-use spice mixes, ready-to-eat vegetable seeds, and spice mixtures such as minced meat. Most of them consist of salt!

Traditional spice mixes such as meat, minced meat, and fish herbs contain salt. But there are also variants without salt for sale: you can often find them in the diet section of the supermarket.

However, the healthiest choice is to prepare **the herb seasoning** yourself with the following dried spices: garlic, basil, oregano, chili, ginger, cinnamon, thyme, and paprika.

Add a tablespoon of each spice to a glass jar and mix well. To preserve the flavor, close the jar and store it in a dry place.

You can change the quantity of each spice according to taste and safely use this mixture to add flavor to vegetables, meat, fish, eggs, and soups.

Eat Less Salty Bread Meals

Each slice of bread contains 0.35 grams of salt. Your salt intake decreases if you choose bread without salt. Bread without salt must be ordered from the bakery or baked yourself.

You also eat less salt if you choose spreads that contain less salt. The siege below has less salt than 1 slice of regular 48+ Gouda cheese or 1 portion of normally salted meats:

- Cheese with less salt (25% or 33% less salt)
- Emmental or Gruyere cheese
- Mon Chou, cottage cheese
- Mozzarella
- Swiss stray cheese
- Slightly salted meats: roast beef, slightly salted smoked meat, fricandeau, turkey breast, chicken breast
- Peanut butter
- Dairy spread
- Sandwich spread, vegetable spread
- Fruit: strawberry, apple/pear slices, banana slices
- Raw vegetables: radish, cress, cucumber slices
- Sweet toppings, such as jam

Have Someone Else Cook (Sometimes)

Do you want to or cannot cook without salt? Then there are several other good options. Do not opt for ready-made meals from the supermarket, the butcher, or the greengrocer. These contain a lot of salt. Below are some good alternatives.

- Open table

Many nursing homes offer residents the option of eating a hot meal for a fee. Diet meals are possible. You must be able to come to the nursing home yourself.

• Meals on Wheels

Table-cover-you is a service for the elderly and the long-term sick. You will receive the complete main meals delivered to your home. That can be a hot or cooled meal you need to heat. Diet meals are possible. Ask about the table at the home care institution in your municipality.

• Frozen meals at home

Some organizations deliver frozen meals to order on demand. Diet meals are often also possible.

Tips Against Food Infections

Good hygiene is always important, even with food that looks good, smells good, and tastes great. Because that too can contain bacteria that make you sick.

- Only eat cooked foods
- Avoid cross-contamination
- Keep prepared products limited
- Avoid products with listeria bacteria
- Be careful with raw products and soft ice cream
- If you are going on holiday abroad, then additional measures apply. The simpler the circumstances and the warmer the climate, the greater the chance that you will contract a food infection.

Only Eat Cooked Foods

Make sure that meat, chicken, and egg are well-cooked before you eat them. The high temperature at which food cooks also kills bacteria.

Avoid Cross-Contamination

During cooking, avoid any contact between raw foods and prepared foods (especially meat, fish, and chicken). Otherwise, you contaminate a cooked dish with new bacteria. Take a clean dish towel and kitchen towel daily. Wash it at 60°C.

Do Not Store Prepared Products for Too Long

You can store prepared products in the fridge for a maximum of 24 hours, provided it is 5°C or cooler in the fridge. If the temperature is higher, the food cannot be stored for as long.

Avoid Raw Products and Soft Ice Cream

Avoid products from raw fish and raw meat, such as shrimp and tartar, and products with raw egg (such as desserts and meringues) and with soft ice cream.

Chapter 3. Foods in Your Pantry

Foods to Eat and Foods to Avoid with Kidney Disease

Some nutrients should be limited in the renal diet, e.g., phosphorus, potassium, and thus any foods that contain high amounts of these should be taken only in low amounts and not on a daily basis. The foods that should be limited are:

- Bananas
- Avocadoes
- Beetroots
- Dried beans
- Dried fruit
- Mangos
- Melons
- Molasses
- Nuts and seeds
- Oranges
- Parsnips
- Spinach
- Potatoes
- Fish
- Low-Fat Yogurt

Be attentive! Following foods have a high amount of sodium, and their consumption should be limited or totally avoided:

- Salty snacks, e.g., pretzels, potato chips, packed popcorn, etc.
- Savory pies, e.g., cheese pies, sausage rolls, and Greek spinach pies
- Processed meats, e.g., luncheon meat, salami, sausages
- Pickled foods in salt brine
- Condiments, e.g., ketchup, mustard, and mayo
- Soy sauce
- Canned soups and sauces

Potassium

Potassium is an important mineral, but higher or lower levels of potassium are harmful to the body. People with chronic kidney disease should maintain ideal potassium levels through a diet. Your per-day potassium intake should be between 2,000 and 2,500 mg.

Sodium

Sodium is an important mineral, but higher or lower levels of Sodium are harmful to the body. People with chronic kidney disease should maintain ideal Sodium levels through a diet. Your per-day Sodium intake should be between 2,000 and 2,500 mg.

Phosphorous

Phosphorous is an important mineral, but higher or lower levels of phosphorous are harmful to the body. People with chronic kidney disease should maintain ideal phosphorous levels through a diet. Your per-day phosphorous intake should be between 800 and 1000 mg.

Kidney-Friendly Dairy Alternatives

- Almond milk
- Rice milk
- Coconut milk

Kidney-Friendly Vegetables

- Cabbage, green/red
- Carrots
- Cauliflower
- Corn
- Cucumber
- Eggplant
- Celery
- Chiles
- Chives
- Arugula
- Asparagus
- Bean sprouts
- Beets, canned
- Ginger root
- Radishes
- Vegetables, mixed
- Green beans
- Lettuce
- Onions

Kidney-Friendly Fruits

- Apple juice
- Apples
- Applesauce
- Cranberries
- Cranberry juice
- Blackberries
- Cherries
- Cranberry sauce
- Grapefruit
- Grapefruit juice
- Grapes
- Figs, fresh
- Fruit cocktail
- Macadamia Nuts
- Pears, canned
- Pineapple
- Lemon
- Lime Peaches
- Plums
- Tangerines
- Raspberries
- Strawberries
- Watermelon

Foods to be consumed in moderate quantities

- Pita bread
- Pretzels, unsalted
- Rice
- Hamburger
- Crackers, unsalted
- Tortillas
- Cereals that are low in sodium, potassium, and phosphorus (check the label)
- Honey

- Jam
- Jelly
- Tofu
- Eggs

Meat and Fish to be consumed in moderate quantities

- Pork
- Turkey
- Beef
- Chicken
- Cod
- Haddock
- Plaice
- Tuna
- Lamb
- Veal

Fats to be consumed in moderate quantities

- Trans-fat free Margarine
- Canola oil
- Nondairy creamers
- Olive oil
- Corn oil

Chapter 4. Easy 5-Weeks Meal Plan

Week 1 plan

Days	Breakfast	Lunch	Snack	Dinner
Day 1	Egg fried rice	Chicken with garlic sauce	Fresh berries	Fish Tacos
Day 2	Italian Apple Fritters	Salmon and Pesto Salad	Coconut Mandarin Salad	Thai Tofu Broth+ Sweet Rice Salad
Day 3	Egg in a Hole	Fish Shakshuka	Almond Caramel Corn	Elegant Veggie Tortillas
Day 4	Apple and Zucchini Bread	Fish Chili with Lentils	Spiced Pretzels	Roasted Cod with Plums+ Lemon Peppers Salad
Day 5	Mushroom and Red Pepper Omelet	Creamy Mushroom Pasta	Tuna Deep	Chili Tofu Noodles+ Healthy Italian Pinzimonio
Day 6	Parmesan Zucchini Frittata	Stuffed Bell Peppers	Cream Dipped Cucumbers	Mango Tilapia Fillets+ Fresh Salad
Day 7	Cottage Cheese Pancakes	Cabbage Rolls Made with Chicken	Cranberry Pecan Salad	Paprika Pork Soup+ Grilled Squash

Week 2 Plan

Days	Breakfast	Lunch	Snack	Dinner
Day 1	Pumpkin Bread	Fish Tacos	Berry Ice Cream	Turkey and Apple Curry
Day 2	Crunchy Potato Croquettes	Tilapia Ceviche	Blueberry Peach Crisp	Broccoli Steaks
Day 3	Vegetarian Summer Rolls	Spicy Lime Shrimp	Cherry Coffee Cake	Beef and Three Pepper Stew
Day 4	Sour Cream and Apple Bread	Couscous with Vegetable	Fruity Peach Crisp Dump	Cajun Crab
Day 5	Strawberry Bread	Seafood Casserole	Gingersnap Cookies	Chunky Beef and Potato Slow Roast
Day 6	Zucchini Bread	Turkey Breast with Cranberry Gravy	Lemon Icebox Pie	Roasted Cod with Plums
Day 7	Asparagus Bacon Hash	Lettuce Seafood Wraps	Strawberry Pavlova	Chicken Soup + Sautéed Green Beans

Week 3 Plan

Days	Breakfast	Lunch	Snack	Dinner
Day 1	Egg White and Pepper Omelet	Chinese Beef Wraps	Seafood Croquettes	Asparagus Quiche+ Zucchini Eggplant with Cheese
Day 2	Turkey Sausage	Sticky Pulled Beef Open Sandwich	Cereal Munch	Sautéed Green Beans
Day 3	Italian Apple Fritters	Fried Scallops in Heavy Cream	Spiced Pretzels	Parsley Root Veg Stew
Day 4	Tofu and Mushroom Scramble	Chicken Lasagna with White Sauce	Italian Tiramisu Cheesecake	Couscous with Vegetable
Day 5	Egg Fried Rice	Mediterranean Vegetable Soup	Chocolate Pie Shell	Chili Mussels+ Eggplant French Fries
Day 6	Cottage Cheese Pancakes	Sage Salmon Fillet	Carrot Corn Bread	Chicken in Herb Sauce+ Curried Veggie Stir-Fry
Day 7	Lemon and Berry Bread	Fish Chili with Lentils	Chocolate Beet Cake	Thai Tofu Broth

Week 4 Plan

Days	Breakfast	Lunch	Snack	Dinner
Day 1	Asparagus Bacon Hash	Beef Stew	Cranberry Pecan Salad	Delicious Vegetarian Lasagna+ Fresh Salad
Day 2	Spicy Corn Bread	Red Pepper and Brie Soup	Sweet Popped Corn	Pork Loins with Leeks+ Healthy Italian Pinzimonio
Day 3	Cajun Stuffed Peppers	Grill Thyme Corn on the Cob	Seafood Croquettes	Vegetarian Quinoa Chilli
Day 4	Platter Zucchini	Oregano Salmon with Crunchy Crust	Strawberry Whipped Cream Cake	Stuffed Bell Peppers
Day 5	Stuffed Lemon and Broccoli	Turkey and Lemongrass Soup	Coconut Mandarin Salad	Ginger Shrimp with Snow Peas
Day 6	Apple Oatmeal Crunch	Lettuce Seafood Wraps	Apple Oatmeal Crunchy	Grilled Skirt Steak+ Fresh Salad
Day 7	Tofu and Mushroom Scramble	Poached Halibut in Lemon Sauce	Berry Ice Cream	Broccoli-Onion Latkes

Week 5 Plan

Days	Breakfast	Lunch	Snack	Dinner
Day 1	Italian Apple Fritters	Spicy Lamb Curry	Blueberry Peach Crisp	Ginger Glazed Carrots
Day 2	Zucchini Bread	4-Ingredients Salmon Fillet	Cream Dipped Cucumbers	Apple Spice Pork Chops
Day 3	Strawberry Bread	Sweet Sour Chicken	Fruity Peach Crisp Dump	Salmon Baked in Foil with Fresh Thyme
Day 4	Sour Cream and Apple Bread	Vegetarian Summer Rolls	Cereal Munch	Chicken and Dumplings
Day 5	Cajun Stuffed Peppers	Fajitas from Turkey	Frozen Lemon Dessert	Cajun Catfish+ Healthy Italian Pinzimonio
Day 6	Crunchy Potato Croquettes	Sardine Fish Cakes	Tuna Deep	Chinese Tempeh Stir Fry+ Sautéed Green Beans
Day 7	Egg Fried Rice	Onion Soup	Falafel Balls	Cabbage Stuffed Mushrooms+Sweet Rice Salad

Chapter 5. Breakfast

Bacon and Egg Tortilla

Diabetes-friendly recipe
Preparation Time: 10 minutes
Cooking Time: 8 minutes
Servings: 2

Ingredients:
- 1 flour tortilla, about 6-inches
- 1/3 cup bacon, chopped
- 1 egg

Directions:
⇒ Take a medium-sized skillet pan, place it over medium heat and when hot, add bacon and cook for 5 minutes.
⇒ When the meat has cooked, drain the excess fat, whisk an egg, pour it into the pan, stir until combined, and cook for 3 minutes, or until eggs have cooked.
⇒ Spoon egg onto the tortilla and then serve.

Nutrition Facts per Serving:
Calories: 337 kcals, **Carbohydrates:** 11 g, **Protein:** 12 g, **Fat:** 27 g, **Sodium:** 460 mg, **Potassium:** 359 mg, **Phosphorus:** 193 mg

Cottage Cheese Pancakes

Diabetes- friendly recipe
Preparation Time: 10 minutes
Cooking Time: 50 minutes
Servings: 4

Ingredients:
- 3 cups fresh raspberries, sliced
- ½ cup all-purpose white flour
- 1 cup cottage cheese, softened
- 3 tablespoons unsalted butter, melted
- 2 eggs, beaten
- 2 egg whites

Directions:
⇒ Crack eggs and egg whites in a medium-sized bowl, add flour, cheese, and butter, and whisk until combined.
⇒ Take a medium-high frying pan, grease it with butter and when hot, pour in prepared batter, ¼ cup of batter per pancake, spread the batter into a 4-inch pancake, and cook for 3 minutes per side until browned.
⇒ When done, transfer pancakes onto a plate; cook more pancakes in the same manner, and, when done, serve each pancake with ½ sliced raspberries.

Nutrition Facts per Serving :
Calories: 272 kcals, **Carbohydrates:** 25g, **Protein:** 14g, **Fat:** 14g, **Sodium:** 262mg, **Potassium:** 272mg, **Phosphorus:** 182mg

Egg in a Hole

Vegetarian-friendly recipe
Preparation Time: 5 minutes
Cooking Time: 5 minutes
Servings: 1

Ingredients:
- 1 slice white bread
- ¼ teaspoon lemon pepper seasoning, salt-free
- 1 egg
- 1 teaspoon Parmesan cheese, grated

Directions:
⇒ Prepare the bread by making a hole in the middle: use a cookie cutter for cutting out the center.
⇒ Brush the slice with oil on both sides, then take a medium-sized skillet pan, place it over medium heat and when hot, add bread slice in it, crack the egg in the center of the slice, and sprinkle with lemon pepper seasoning.
⇒ Cook the egg for 2 minutes, then carefully flip it along with the slice and continue cooking for an additional 2 minutes.
⇒ Sprinkle cheese on the egg, let it melt, then slide the egg onto a plate; serve straight away.

Nutrition Facts per Serving :
Calories: 141 kcals, **Carbohydrates:** 13g, **Protein:** 6 g, **Fat:** 9 g, **Sodium:** 330 mg, **Potassium:** 122 mg, **Phosphorus:** 137 mg

German Pancakes

Preparation Time: 10 minutes
Cooking Time: 15 minutes
Servings: 4

Ingredients:
- 5 tablespoons all-purpose flour
- ¼ teaspoon vanilla extract, unsweetened
- 2 tablespoons white sugar
- 1 cup milk, low-fat
- 2 eggs
- ½ cup cream cheese, softened
- 1 tablespoon fruit jam per serving, sugar-free

Directions:
⇒ Prepare the batter by taking a medium-sized bowl, add flour in it along with sugar, stir until mixed, whisk in eggs until blended, and then whisk in vanilla and milk until smooth.
⇒ Take a skillet pan, about 8 inches, spray it with oil and when hot, add 3 tablespoons of the prepared batter, tilt the pan to spread the batter evenly, and cook for 45 seconds, or until the bottom is browned.
⇒ Flip the pancake, continue cooking for 45 seconds until the other side is browned, and when done, transfer the pancake to a plate.
⇒ Cook nine more pancakes in the same manner and, when done, spread 2 tablespoons of cream cheese on one side of the pancake, fold it, and then serve with 1 tablespoon of fruit jam.

Nutrition Facts per Serving :
Calories: 120 kcals, **Carbohydrates:** 10 g, **Protein:** 4 g, **Fat:** 2 g, **Sodium:** 39 mg, **Potassium:** 73 mg, **Phosphorus:** 76 mg

Mushroom and Red Pepper Omelet

Vegetarian-friendly Recipe
Preparation Time: *5 minutes*
Cooking Time: *12 minutes*
Servings: 2

Ingredients:
- 2 tablespoons white onion, diced
- ¼ cup sweet red peppers, diced
- ½ cup mushrooms, diced
- ¼ teaspoon ground black pepper
- 1 teaspoon Worcestershire sauce
- 1 egg
- 1 egg white
- 2 tablespoons olive oil
- 2 tablespoons light cream cheese

Directions:
⇒ Take a medium-sized skillet pan, place it over medium heat, and add 1 teaspoon olive oil and when it melts, add onions and mushrooms and cook for 5 minutes or until onions are tender.
⇒ Stir in red pepper, then transfer vegetables to a plate and set aside until needed.
⇒ Crack the egg and the egg white in a bowl, add Worcestershire sauce, and whisk until combined.
⇒ Return skillet pan over medium heat, add remaining olive oil, and when it melts, pour in the egg mixture, and cook for 2 minutes, or until omelet is partially cooked.
⇒ Then top cooked vegetables on one side of the omelet, top with light cream cheese, and continue cooking until the omelet is cooked completely.
⇒ When done, remove the pan from the heat, cover the filling of the omelet by folding the other half of the omelet, sprinkle it with black pepper, and then divide the omelet into two.
⇒ Serve straight away.

Nutrition Facts per Serving :
Calories: 213 kcals, **Carbohydrates:** 5g, **Protein:** 7 , **Fat:** 18g, **Sodium:** 140mg, **Potassium:** 252mg, **Phosphorus:** 101mg

Apple and Zucchini Bread

Vegetarian-friendly
Preparation Time: 15 minutes
Cooking Time: 50 minutes
Servings: 6

Ingredients:
Loaves:
- 2 cups zucchini, grated
- 3 ½ cups and 2 tablespoons all-purpose white flour
- 1 cup apples, chopped
- 1 ½ teaspoons baking soda
- ½ cup honey
- ½ teaspoon herb seasoning
- 3 teaspoons ground cinnamon
- ¾ cup Splenda® brown sugar blend
- 1 teaspoon vanilla extract, unsweetened
- ½ cup olive oil
- 2 eggs + 2 egg whites

Directions:
⇒ Switch on the oven, then set it to 350°F and let it preheat.

⇒ Meanwhile, take two 9-by-5 inches loaf pans, spray them with oil, sprinkle with 2 tablespoons of flour, and set aside until needed.
⇒ Crack eggs in a large bowl, add vanilla, eggs, oil, honey, and ¾ cup brown sugar, and whisk until combined.
⇒ Take another large bowl, add remaining flour in it, stir in baking soda, 2 tablespoons cinnamon, and salt until mixed, and then gradually stir the flour mixture into egg mixture until incorporated. Don't over-mix.
⇒ Then fold in grated zucchini and chopped apples until mixed, distribute the batter evenly between the two prepared loaf pans and bake in the heated oven for 50 minutes.
⇒ Cut each loaf into eighteen slices, each about ½-inch thick, and then serve.

Nutrition Facts per Serving :
Calories: 619 kcals, **Carbohydrates:** 97g, **Protein:** 11g, **Fat:** 10g, **Sodium:** 81mg, **Potassium:** 350mg, **Phosphorus:** 180 mg

Spicy Corn Bread

Diabetes-friendly recipe
Preparation Time: 15 minutes
Cooking Time: 30 minutes
Servings: 4

Ingredients
o ½ cup scallions, chopped
o ¼ teaspoon minced garlic
o ¼ cup carrots, grated
o 1 cup cornmeal
o 1 cup all-purpose white flour
o 2 teaspoons baking powder
o ¼ teaspoon ground black pepper
o 1 tablespoon white sugar
o 1 teaspoon red chili powder
o 1 egg
o 2 tablespoons canola oil
o 1 egg white
o 1 cup of rice milk

Directions:
⇒ Switch on the oven, then set it to 400°F and let it preheat.
⇒ Meanwhile, take a large bowl, add cornmeal and flour, and then stir in black pepper, red chili powder, baking powder, and sugar until combined.
⇒ Take another large bowl, add egg and egg white, whisk in oil and milk until blended, and then gradually whisk this mixture into the flour mixture until incorporated.

⇒ Add carrots, scallions, and garlic, stir until just mixed, then take an 8-inches baking pan, grease it with oil, pour the prepared batter in it, and bake for 30 minutes until bread is firm and the top has turned golden-brown.
⇒ When done, let the bread cool for 10 minutes in the pan, then take it out; cut the bread into eight pieces, each about 2-by-4 inches, and serve.

Nutrition Facts per Serving :
Calories: 267 kcals, **Carbohydrates:** 45g, **Protein:** 6g, **Fat:** 7g, **Sodium:** 217mg, **Potassium:** 141mg, **Phosphorus:** 218mg

Pumpkin Bread

Vegetarian-friendly recipe
Preparation Time: 20 minutes
Cooking Time: 45 minutes
Servings: 6

Ingredients
o 3 ½ cups all-purpose white flour
o 2 cups pumpkin
o 1 teaspoon ginger powder
o ½ teaspoon baking powder
o 1 teaspoon cinnamon
o 1 teaspoon herb seasoning (see recipe)
o 1 cup white sugar
o ½ cup olive oil
o ¾ cup water
o 1 egg
o 3 egg whites

Directions:
⇒ Switch on the oven, then set it to 350°F, and let it preheat.
⇒ Meanwhile, take a large bowl, crack eggs in it, add pumpkin, sugar, oil, and water and whisk until beaten.
⇒ Gradually beat in flour, baking soda, ginger, cinnamon, and salt until smooth, distribute the batter evenly between three loaf pans and then bake for 45 minutes until the top has turn golden-brown and loaves pass the skewer test (if the skewer comes out clean from the center of the bread).
⇒ When done, let the loaves cool in the pan for 10 minutes, then take them out from the pan and cool them for 20 minutes on the wire rack.
⇒ Cut each loaf into twelve slices and then serve two slices per person.

Nutrition Facts per Serving :
Calories: 570 kcals, **Carbohydrates:** 86g, **Protein:** 11g, **Fat:** 20g, **Sodium:** 85mg, **Potassium:** 287mg, **Phosphorus:** 123mg

Crunchy Potato Croquettes

Vegetarian-friendly recipe
Preparation Time: 15 minutes
Cooking Time: 20 minutes
Servings: 4

Ingredients:
- 4 medium "leached" potato, cooked and peeled
- 1 tablespoon butter
- 1 tablespoon rice milk
- 1 tablespoon pepper
- 1 beaten egg
- 1 cup white breadcrumbs
- 2 tablespoon canola oil

Directions:
⇒ Mash potatoes with milk, butter, and pepper.
⇒ Form cooled potatoes into balls with your hands.
⇒ Dip balls in beaten egg.
⇒ Next, roll balls in breadcrumbs.
⇒ Then place balls in a hot oiled skillet and fry until golden brown.

Nutrition Facts per Serving:
Calories: 460 kcal, **Carbohydrates:** 73,33 g, **Protein:** 12 g, **Fat:** 13 g, **Sodium:** 381 mg, **Potassium:** 1039 mg, **Phosphorus:** 228 mg

Vegetarian Summer Rolls

Vegetarian-friendly recipe
Preparation Time: 5 Minutes
Cooking Time: 20 minutes
Servings: 4

Ingredients:
- 1-ounce rice vermicelli noodles
- 2 zucchinis shredded
- 2 carrots shredded
- 2 shallots finely chopped
- 2 small cucumbers peeled and diced
- ¾ cup fresh basil chopped
- ½ cup fresh cilantro chopped
- 12 spring roll wrappers

Dipping Sauce:
- 2 tablespoons honey
- 1/4 cup rice vinegar
- 2 fresh red chilies

Directions:
⇒ Place honey, vinegar, and 2 tablespoons of water in a saucepan and boil gently.
⇒ Remove from heat, add chilies, and set aside.
⇒ In a large bowl, combine all rest of the ingredients (except wrappers).
⇒ Place a moistened wrapper on a work surface.
⇒ Put a spoonful of filling in the center and fold to encase, bringing corner to corner.
⇒ Fold in sides and roll up tightly. Brush end with water to seal.
⇒ Repeat until all filling is used.
⇒ Serve with dipping sauce.

Nutrition Facts per Serving:
Calories: 204 kcals, **Carbohydrates:** 45g, **Protein:** 6g, **Fat:** 1g, **Sodium:** 212mg, **Potassium:** 665mg, **Phosphorus:** 126mg

Sour Cream and Apple Bread

Diabetes-friendly recipe
Preparation Time: 20 minutes
Cooking Time: 55 minutes
Servings: 4

Ingredients:
- 1 cup diced apple
- 1 ¾ cups all-purpose white flour
- ¾ teaspoon baking powder
- ½ cup white sugar
- ¼ teaspoon baking soda
- ½ teaspoon ground cinnamon
- ¼ cup canola oil
- 2 egg whites
- ¾ cup applesauce, unsweetened
- ¾ cup sour cream, reduced-fat
- 6 tablespoons water

Directions:
⇒ Preheat oven to 350°F.
⇒ Meanwhile, take a large bowl, add flour to it and then stir in baking soda and powder and cinnamon until mixed.
⇒ Take a separate bowl, add oil in it, beat in sugar until well combined, then gradually beat in flour mixture, egg whites, and applesauce until incorporated and fold in apples and sour cream until just mixed. Take an 8.5-by-4.75 inches loaf pan, grease it with oil, pour the batter in it and then bake for 55 minutes until the top has turned golden-brown and the loaf passes the skewer test (if the skewer comes out clean from the center of the bread).
⇒ When done, let the loaf cool in the pan for 10 minutes, then take it out from the pan, and cool them for 20 minutes on the wire rack.
⇒ Cut the loaf into ten slices, and then serve.

Nutrition Facts per Serving:
Calories: 330 kcals, **Carbohydrates:** 49g, **Protein:** 6g, **Fat:** 12g, **Sodium:** 190mg, **Potassium:** 129mg, **Phosphorus:** 81mg

Strawberry Bread

Diabetes-friendly recipe
Preparation Time: 10 minutes
Cooking Time: 50 minutes
Serving: 4

Ingredients:
- 2 cups all-purpose white flour
- 1 teaspoon baking soda
- ¼ teaspoon ground cinnamon
- 2 cups white sugar
- 1 cup canola oil
- 2 eggs
- 3 cups fresh strawberries, chopped
- 6 tablespoons water

Directions:
⇒ Preheat the oven to 350°F.
⇒ Crack eggs in a medium bowl, beat in oil until incorporated, and then stir in berries until mixed.
⇒ Take a separate large bowl, add flour in it along with remaining ingredients, stir until mixed, then make a well in the center, pour in egg batter, and mix well until blended. Don't over-mix.
⇒ Take two 9-by-5 inches loaf pans, distribute the batter evenly between them, and then bake for 60 minutes until the top has turned golden-brown, and loaves pass the skewer test (if the skewer comes out clean from the center of the bread).
⇒ When done, let the loaves cool in the pan for 15 minutes, then take them out from the pan, and cool them for an additional 20 minutes on the wire rack.
⇒ Cut each loaf into slices, and then serve.

Nutrition Facts per Serving:
Calories: 443 kcals, **Carbohydrates:** 61g, **Protein:** 7g, **Fat:** 20g, **Sodium:** 217mg, **Potassium:** 248mg, **Phosphorus:** 127mg

Zucchini Bread

Vegetarian-friendly recipe
Preparation Time: 20 minutes
Cooking Time: 60 minutes
Servings: 6

Ingredients:
- 3 cups zucchini, grated
- 2 cups all-purpose white flour
- 1 teaspoon herb seasoning (see recipe)
- 1 ½ teaspoons baking soda
- ¼ cup Splenda® granulated sweetener
- 1 ½ teaspoons pumpkin pie spice
- 2 tablespoons lemon juice
- 1 teaspoon vanilla extract, unsweetened
- 3 tablespoons honey
- 4 tablespoons olive oil
- 4 eggs
- ¾ cup applesauce, unsweetened

Directions:
⇒ Preheat the oven to 350°F.
⇒ Meanwhile, take a large bowl, add flour to it and then stir in herb seasoning (see recipe), Splenda®, baking soda, and pumpkin pie spice until mixed.
⇒ Take a separate bowl, crack eggs in it, beat until blended, stir in remaining ingredients until incorporated, and then stir this mixture gradually into flour mixture until combined. Don't over-mix.
⇒ Take two 8.5-by-4.5 inches loaf pans, distribute the batter evenly between them, and then bake for 60 minutes until the top has turned golden-brown, and loaves pass the skewer test (if the skewer comes out clean from the center of the bread).
⇒ When done, let the loaves cool in the pan for 10 minutes, then take them out from the pan, and cool them for an additional 20 minutes on the wire rack.
⇒ Cut each loaf into twelve slices, and then serve.

Nutrition Facts per Serving:
Calories: 321 kcals, **Carbohydrates:** 47g, **Protein:** 8g, **Fat:** 12g, **Sodium:** 78mg, **Potassium:** 326mg, **Phosphorus:** 151mg

Blistered Beans and Almond

Vegetarian-friendly recipe
Preparation Time: 10 minutes
Cooking Time: 20 minutes
Servings: 4

Ingredients:
- 1 pound fresh green beans, ends trimmed
- 1 ½ tablespoon olive oil
- ½ tablespoon herb seasoning (see recipe)
- 1 ½ tablespoon fresh dill, minced
- 1 lemon, juice
- ¼ cup crushed almonds

Directions:
⇒ Preheat your oven to 400°F.
⇒ Add in the green beans with your olive oil.
⇒ Then spread them in one single layer on a large-sized sheet pan.
⇒ Roast for 10 minutes, and stir nicely, then roast for another 8–10 minutes.
⇒ Remove it from the oven, and keep stirring in the lemon juice alongside the dill.
⇒ Top it with crushed almonds, some herb seasoning and serve.

Nutrition Facts per Serving:
Calories: 146 kcals, **Carbohydrates:** 11g, **Protein:** 5g, **Fat:** 11g, **Sodium:** 57mg, **Potassium:** 329mg, **Phosphorus:** 95mg

Lemon and Broccoli Platter

Vegetarian-friendly recipe
Preparation Time: 10 minutes
Cooking Time: 15 minutes
Servings: 4

Ingredients:
- 2 heads broccoli, separated into florets
- 2 teaspoons extra virgin olive oil
- 1 teaspoon herb seasoning (see recipe)
- ½ teaspoon black pepper
- 1 garlic clove, minced
- ½ teaspoon lemon juice

Directions:
⇒ Preheat your oven to 400°F.
⇒ Bring a large pot of water to a boil and drop in the broccoli florets.
⇒ Boil the broccoli for 5 minutes. Remove, and drain.
⇒ Take a large-sized bowl and add broccoli florets.
⇒ Drizzle olive oil, and season with pepper, herb seasoning, and garlic.
⇒ Spread the broccoli out in a single even layer on a baking sheet.
⇒ Bake for 15–20 minutes until fork tender.
⇒ Squeeze lemon juice on top.
⇒ Serve and enjoy!

Nutrition Facts per Serving:
Calories: 49 kcals, **Carbohydrates:** 6 g, **Protein:** 3 g, **Fat:** 3 g, **Sodium:** 75 mg, **Potassium:** 246 mg, **Phosphorus:** 52 mg

Egg White and Pepper Omelet

Diabetes-friendly recipe
Preparation Time: 5 minutes
Cooking Time: 5 minutes
Servings: 2

Ingredients:
- 4 egg whites, lightly beaten
- 1 red bell pepper, diced
- 1 teaspoon paprika
- 2 tablespoon olive oil
- ½ teaspoon pepper

Directions:

⇒ In a shallow non-stick frying pan (around 8 inches), heat the olive oil, and sauté the bell peppers until softened.
⇒ Add egg whites and paprika and fold the edges into the fluid center with a spatula, and let omelet cook until eggs are fully opaque and solid.
⇒ Season with pepper and serve.

Nutrition Facts per Serving:
Calories: 176 kcals, **Carbohydrates:** 5 g, **Protein:** 7 g, **Fat:** 14 g, **Sodium:** 99 mg, **Potassium:** 254 mg, **Phosphorus:** 29 mg

Turkey Sausage

Diabetes-friendly recipe
Preparation Time: 5 minutes
Cooking Time: 6 minutes
Servings: 6

Ingredients:
- 1 pound lean ground turkey
- 1 tablespoon fennel seed
- ¼ tablespoon garlic powder
- ¼ tablespoon onion powder
- 2 tablespoon vegetable oil
- ¼ tablespoon pepper

Directions:
⇒ Combine all the ingredients apart from the vegetable oil in a mixing bowl.
⇒ Form into long and flat (around 4 inch-long) patties.
⇒ Heat the vegetable oil in a medium frying pan.
⇒ Add 3–4 patties at a time and cook for approximately 3 minutes on each side. Repeat until you cook all the patties.
⇒ Serve warm.

Nutrition Facts per Serving:
Calories: 276 kcals, **Carbohydrates:** 2 g, **Protein:** 20 g, **Fat:** 22 g, **Sodium:** 208 mg, **Potassium:** 272 mg, **Phosphorus:** 215 mg

Italian Apple Fritters

Vegetarian-friendly recipe
Preparation Time: 5 minutes
Cooking Time: 8 minutes
Servings: 4

Ingredients:
- 2 large apples, seeded, peeled, and thickly sliced in round circles

- 3 tablespoons corn flour
- ½ tablespoon water
- 2 teaspoons honey
- ½ tablespoon cinnamon
- Corn oil

Directions:
⇒ Combine the corn flour, water, and 1 teaspoon honey to make your batter in a small bowl.
⇒ Deep the apple rounds into the corn flour mix.
⇒ Heat enough vegetable oil to cover half of the pan's surface over medium to high heat.
⇒ Add the apple rounds into the pan and cook until golden brown.
⇒ Transfer into a shallow dish with paper towels on top, and sprinkle with a bit of cinnamon.

Nutrition Facts per Serving:
Calories: 110 kcals, **Carbohydrates:** 6 g, **Protein:** 1 g, **Fat:** 4 g, **Sodium:** 1 mg, **Potassium:** 97 mg, **Phosphorus:** 14 mg

Tofu and Mushroom Scramble

Vegetarian-friendly recipe
Preparation Time: 5 minutes
Cooking Time: 4 minutes
Servings: 4

Ingredients:
- 1 cup sliced white mushrooms
- ½ cup medium-firm tofu, crumbled
- 2 tablespoon chopped shallots
- ¾ tablespoon turmeric
- 2 tablespoon cumin
- ½ tablespoon smoked paprika
- 1 teaspoon pepper
- 2 tablespoons sunflower oil

Directions:
⇒ Take a non-stick frying pan and heat the oil.
⇒ Sauté the sliced mushrooms with the shallots until softened (around 3–4 minutes) over medium to high heat.
⇒ Add the tofu pieces and sprinkle in the spices.
⇒ Stir lightly until tofu and mushrooms are nicely combined together.
⇒ Serve warm.

Nutrition Facts per Serving:
Calories: 113 kcals, **Carbohydrates:** 6 g, **Protein:** 4 g, **Fat:** 9 g, **Sodium:** 24 mg, **Potassium:** 284 mg, **Phosphorus:** 52 mg

Egg Fried Rice

Gluten-free
Preparation Time: 10 minutes
Cooking Time: 20 minutes
Servings: 4

Ingredients:
- 1 teaspoon olive oil
- 1 tablespoon grated peeled fresh ginger
- 1 teaspoon minced garlic
- 1 cup chopped carrots
- 1 scallion, white and green parts, chopped
- 2 tablespoons chopped fresh cilantro
- 2 cups cooked rice
- 1 tablespoon low-sodium soy sauce
- 1 egg, lightly beaten

Directions:
⇒ In a large non-stick frying pan and heat the olive oil medium heat.
⇒ Add the ginger and garlic, and sauté until softened, for about 3 minutes.
⇒ Add the carrots, scallion, and cilantro, and sauté until tender, for about 5 minutes.
⇒ Stir in the rice and soy sauce, and sauté until the rice is heated through about 5 minutes.
⇒ Move the rice over to one side of the skillet and pour the egg into the empty space.
⇒ Scramble the egg, and then mix them into the rice.
⇒ Serve hot.

Nutrition Facts per Serving:
Calories: 164 kcals, **Carbohydrates:** 30 g, **Protein:** 4 g, **Fat:** 3 g,
Sodium: 60 mg, **Potassium:** 179 mg, **Phosphorus:** 70 mg

Lemon and Berry Bread

Diabetes-friendly recipe
Preparation Time: 10 minutes
Cooking Time: 54 minutes
Servings: 6

Ingredients:
- 2 cups blueberries, fresh
- 1 cup all-purpose white flour
- 1 teaspoon baking powder
- 1/4 cup honey
- 2 tablespoons of granulated sugar
- 1/3 cup corn oil
- 2 tablespoons lemon zest, grated
- 2 tablespoons lemon extract, unsweetened
- ½ cup lemon juice
- 2 eggs
- ½ cup milk, skimmed

Directions:
⇒ Preheat the oven to 350°F.
⇒ Meanwhile, take a large bowl, add 1 cup of flour, the baking powder and stir well.
⇒ Take another bowl, add oil and beat in egg white, lemon extract, and honey until well combined.
⇒ Then whisk in flour mixture alternating with milk until just mixed (do not over-mix), and fold in lemon zest and berries until combined.
⇒ Take a 9-by-5-3 inches loaf pan, grease it with oil, sprinkle with 1 tablespoon flour, pour in prepared batter in it, and bake for 50 minutes until the top has turned golden-brown and the loaf passes the skewer test (if the skewer comes out clean from the center of the bread).
⇒ Prepare the glaze: in a saucepan over medium heat, add granulated sugar, stir in lemon juice and cook for 4 minutes, or until the sugar has dissolved.
⇒ When the bread has baked, let the loaf cool in the pan for 10 minutes, then take it out poke holes on the top at the 1-inch interval, and pour prepared glaze on the bread. Let it cool for 10 minutes.
⇒ Cut the loaf into ten slices and serve.

Nutrition Facts per Serving:
Calories: 309 kcals, **Carbohydrates:** 42 g, **Protein:** 5 g, **Fat:** 15 g, **Sodium:** 112 mg, **Potassium:** 143 mg, **Phosphorus:** 97 mg

Asparagus Bacon Hash

Vegetarian-friendly recipe
Preparation Time: 10 minutes
Cooking Time: 18 minutes
Servings: 4

Ingredients:
o 2 slices bacon, diced
o 1/2 onion, chopped
o 1 garlic clove, sliced
o 2 lb. asparagus, trimmed and chopped
o Black pepper, to taste
o 1 tablespoons Parmesan, grated
o 4 large eggs
o 1/4 teaspoon red pepper flakes

Directions:
⇒ Add the asparagus and a tablespoon of water to a microwave-proof bowl.
⇒ Cover the veggies and microwave them for 5 minutes until tender.
⇒ Set a suitable non-stick frying pan over moderate heat and layer it with cooking spray.
⇒ Stir in the onion and sauté for 8 minutes, and then add in bacon and garlic.
⇒ Stir for 1 minute, and then add in the asparagus, eggs, and red pepper flakes.
⇒ Reduce the heat to low and cover the vegetables in the pan. Top the eggs with Parmesan cheese.
⇒ Cook for 5 minutes, then slice to serve.

Nutrition Facts per Serving:
Calories: 173 kcals, **Carbohydrates:** 11g, **Protein:** 13g, **Fat:** 10g, **Sodium:** 165mg, **Potassium:** 573mg, **Phosphorus:** 237mg

Parmesan Zucchini Frittata

Vegetarian-friendly recipe
Preparation Time: 10 minutes
Cooking Time: 35 minutes
Servings: 4

Ingredients:
o 1 tablespoon olive oil
o 1 cup yellow onion, sliced
o 3 cups zucchini, chopped
o 2 tablespoons Parmesan cheese, grated
o 2 large eggs
o ½ cup milk, skimmed
o ½ teaspoon black pepper
o ⅛ teaspoon paprika

Directions:
⇒ Preheat the oven to 350°F.
⇒ Grease a 11x7 inches baking tray with cooking spray.
⇒ In a large bowl add eggs, milk, parmesan and stir well.
⇒ Add zucchinis, onion, paprika, pepper and stir gently.
⇒ Pour this mixture into the baking tray and spread it evenly.
⇒ Bake the zucchini casserole for approximately 20 minutes.
⇒ Cut in 4 slices and serve..

Nutrition Facts per Serving:
Calories: 74 kcals, **Carbohydrates:** 8g, **Protein:** 5g, **Fat:** 3g, **Sodium:** 53mg, **Potassium:** 390mg, **Phosphorus:** 122mg

Mexican Baked Beans and Rice

Vegetarian-friendly recipe
Preparation Time: 20 minutes
Cooking Time: 45 minutes
Servings: 4

Ingredients:
o 2 garlic cloves, crushed
o 1 tbsp. cumin

- 1 tbsp. chili powder
- 1 cup chopped poblano pepper
- 1 cup chopped red bell pepper
- Black beans (8-oz, no-salt-added), drained and rinsed
- 6 fresh tomatoes, diced
- ½ lb. chicken breast, skinless, boneless, cubed
- 1 ½ cups cooked white rice

Directions:
- With cooking spray, grease a ¾ shallow casserole, and preheat oven to 400°F.
- Spread cooked rice at the bottom of the casserole. Layer chicken on top of rice.
- Mix well garlic, seasonings, peppers, beans, and tomatoes in a medium bowl. Evenly spread bean mixture on top of chicken. Pop into the oven. Set to bake until cooked for 45 minutes.
- Serve hot.

Nutrition Facts per Serving:
Calories: Calories: 306 kcals, **Carbohydrates:** 36g, **Protein:** 20g, **Fat:** 10g, **Sodium:** 315mg, **Potassium:** 1017mg, **Phosphorus:** 269mg

Quick Thai Chicken and Vegetable Curry

Preparation Time: 10 minutes
Cooking Time: 30 minutes
Servings: 4

Ingredients:
- 1 ½ cups cauliflower florets
- 1 clove garlic, minced
- 1 cup light coconut milk
- 1 cup water
- 1 lb. chicken breasts
- 1 medium bell pepper, julienned
- 1 medium onion, halved and sliced
- 1 tablespoon fresh ginger, minced
- 1 tablespoon lime juice
- 1 tablespoon light brown sugar
- 1 tablespoon red curry paste
- 1 cup baby spinach
- 2 tablespoon corn oil
- 4 lime wedges

Directions:
- Heat oil in a non-stick frying pan over medium heat.
- Sauté the onion and bell pepper for four minutes or until soft.
- Add the ginger, garlic, and curry paste. Mix, then add the chicken. Sauté for two minutes before adding the coconut milk, water, soy sauce and brown sugar.
- Add the cauliflowers and reduce the heat to medium-low.
- Simmer, and stir the mixture occasionally for 20 minutes, until the chicken is cooked through.
- Add the spinach and lime juice and cook for 5 minutes.
- Serve immediately with lime wedges.

Nutrition Facts per Serving:
Calories: 350 kcals, **Carbohydrates:** 13g, **Protein:** 26g, **Fat:** 22 g, **Sodium:** 577mg, **Potassium:** 577mg, **Phosphorus:** 237mg

Cajun Stuffed Peppers

Preparation Time: 10 minutes
Cooking Time: 55 minutes
Servings: 4

Ingredients:
- 2 fresh bell peppers
- 1/2 lb. ground chicken
- 1/4 cup hot water
- 1 medium onion chopped
- 1 cup cooked white rice
- 1/4 tablespoon black pepper
- 1/4 tablespoon lemon pepper
- 1/2 tablespoon dried thyme
- 1 tablespoon minced garlic

Directions:
- Preheat oven to 350°F.
- Bring a large pot of water to a boil and drop in the bell peppers. Blanch them for 5 minutes. Remove, and drain.
- Cut the peppers in half lengthwise, remove the stem and the seeds.
- In a large non-stick shallow pan, cook the ground meat over medium heat for 5 minutes.
- Add the hot water, onions, garlic, and spices.
- Cook for 5 minutes.
- Add rice and stir to combine and cook for 3 minutes. Remove from the heat and stuff the bell

peppers. Put the stuffed peppers on a baking sheet and bake, covered, for 30 minutes.
⇒ Uncover and bake for 10 minutes more.
⇒ Serve hot.

Nutrition Facts per Serving:
Calories: Calories: 155 kcals, **Carbohydrates:** 16g, **Protein:** 12g, **Fat:** 5g, **Sodium:** 174mg, **Potassium:** 475mg, **Phosphorus:** 130mg

Stuffed Zucchinis

Vegetarian-friendly recipe
Preparation Time: 10 minutes
Cooking Time: 55 minutes
Servings: 4

Ingredients:
- 4 large zucchinis
- 2 tablespoons olive oil
- 1 onion, diced
- 1 tablespoon fresh coriander
- 1 tablespoon minced garlic
- 1 teaspoon ground pepper

Directions:
⇒ Preheat oven to 350°F.
⇒ Bring a large pot of water to a boil and drop in the zucchinis. Blanch them for 2 minutes. Remove, and drain.
⇒ Slice zucchini in half, lengthwise, and scoop out insides leaving ¼ inch zucchini on skins. Reserve the insides.
⇒ Place zucchini halves skin-side down on the baking sheet.
⇒ In a large non-stick frying pan warm the oil over medium heat.
⇒ Add the onion and sauté for 5 minutes.
⇒ Add the zucchini inside, the breadcrumbs and the spices. Sauté for 5 minutes.
⇒ Remove from heat, and stuff the zucchini with the mixture.
⇒ Bake covered for 30 minutes, then uncovered for 10 minutes more.
⇒ Serve warm.

Nutrition Facts per Serving:
Calories: 301 kcals, **Carbohydrates:** 44g, **Protein:** 9g, **Fat:** 10g, **Sodium:** 379mg, **Potassium:** 654mg, **Phosphorus:** 163mg

Chapter 6. Soups

Chicken Fajita Soup

Diabetes-friendly recipe
Preparation Time: 5 minutes
Cooking Time: 1 hours 45 minutes
Servings: 4

Ingredients:
- 10 ounces boneless skinless chicken breasts
- 1 teaspoon ground pepper
- 1 onion chopped
- 1 green pepper chopped
- 2 garlic cloves minced
- 1 tablespoon of olive oil
- 6 tomatoes diced
- 2 teaspoons chili powder
- 1 cup chicken broth
- 2 cups water
- ½ tablespoon herb seasoning (see recipe)

Directions:
⇒ Add boneless skinless chicken breasts to a cooking pot and simmer for 1 hour in a cup of chicken broth and 1 cup of water. Season with pepper.
⇒ When the chicken is done, remove from the pot and shred. Keep the leftover broth for the soup.
⇒ In a large non-stick frying pan add 1 tablespoon of olive oil, green pepper, onion, tomatoes, chili powder and sauté for 5 minutes.
⇒ Add the shredded chicken to the cooking pot with the broth, add remaining water and the vegetables.
⇒ Cover and cook for 40 minutes.
⇒ Serve hot and enjoy!

Nutrition Facts per Serving:
Calories: 179 kcals, **Carbohydrates:** 13g, **Protein:** 19 g, **Fat:** 6g, **Sodium:** 607mg, **Potassium:** 821mg, **Phosphorus:** 220mg

Italian Soup

Diabetes-friendly recipe
Preparation Time: 5 minutes
Cooking Time: 55 minutes
Servings: 4

Ingredients:
- 2 tablespoons olive oil
- ¼ cup onion, diced
- 2 celery stalks, chopped
- 2 cloves garlic, minced
- 2 cups riced cauliflower
- 4 tomatoes, diced
- 1 cup zucchinis, diced
- 1 cup carrots, sliced into 1-inch pieces
- 1 cup water
- 2 cups chicken broth
- 1 teaspoon dried oregano
- ½ teaspoon pepper
- 4 teaspoons parmesan for sprinkling

Directions:
⇒ Mix together all the vegetables in a non-stick or glazed clay cooking pot.
⇒ Add the olive oil and sauté for 5 minutes.
⇒ Add the garlic and cook for 1 minute.
⇒ Stir in chicken broth, water, oregano, pepper and simmer for 50 minutes.
⇒ Serve hot with parmesan and enjoy.

Nutrition Facts per Serving:
Calories: 138 kcals, **Carbohydrates:** 14g, **Protein:** 4g, **Fat:** 8g, **Sodium:** 533mg, **Potassium:** 714 mg, **Phosphorus:** 98mg

Cream of Chicken Soup

Diabetes-friendly recipe
Preparation Time: 10 minutes
Cooking Time: 20 minutes
Servings: 4

Ingredients:
- 1 tablespoon olive oil
- 2 onions, diced
- 1 potato, boiled and diced
- 1 large carrot, boiled and diced
- 1 celery stick, diced
- 2 tablespoons plain flour
- 2 cups chicken broth
- 1 cup skimmed milk
- ½ lb cooked chicken
- 4 teaspoons single cream
- ¼ teaspoon freshly ground black pepper

Directions:
⇒ Add the oil in a large non-stick cooking pot and cook the onions, potatoes, carrots and celery gently for about 5 minutes.
⇒ Sprinkle over the flour, and cook over low heat for 5 minutes, stirring all the time. Gradually pour in the broth and the milk, stirring every few minutes and allow to come to the boil.
⇒ Remove from the heat.
⇒ Add the cooked chicken, pepper and simmer for 5 minutes.
⇒ Pour the soup into a food processor or blender in batches and blend until smooth.
⇒ Transfer back into the soup pot and serve with one teaspoon of cream for each serving.

Nutrition Facts per Serving: **Calories:** 248 kcals, **Carbohydrates:** 23g, **Protein:** 21g, **Fat:** 8g, **Sodium:** 539mg, **Potassium:** 608mg, **Phosphorus:** 209mg

Green Chicken Enchilada Soup

Diabetes-friendly recipe
Preparation Time: 5 minutes
Cooking Time: 20 minutes
Servings: 4

Ingredients:
- 1 tablespoon salsa verde
- ½ tablespoon onion powder
- ½ tablespoon garlic powder
- 1 cup skimmed milk
- ½ cup sharp cheddar cheese, shredded
- 1 cup chicken stock
- 1 cup water
- 2 cups cooked chicken, shredded

Directions:
⇒ With a food processor blend all the ingredients except the chicken.
⇒ Simmer for 10 minutes in a cooking pot over medium heat.
⇒ Add cooked the cooked chicken and cook for 15 minutes over low heat.
⇒ Serve and enjoy

Nutrition Facts per Serving:
Calories: 232 kcals, **Carbohydrates:** 5g, **Protein:** 20g, **Fat:** 14g, **Sodium:** 276mg, **Potassium:** 260mg, **Phosphorus:** 225mg.

Beef Stew

Diabetes-friendly recipe
Preparation Time: 10 minutes
Cooking Time: 1 hour
Servings: 4

Ingredients:
- 1 pound Beef Short Rib, thinly sliced
- 1 tablespoon olive oil
- ½ teaspoon Xanthan Gum
- 1 cups beef broth
- 1 cup water
- 4 cloves minced garlic
- 1 onion, diced
- 1 potato, diced
- 1 large carrot, diced
- ¼ teaspoon pepper

Directions:
⇒ Add onions, garlic, and olive oil in a large pan and sauté for 5 minutes.
⇒ Once the onions are soft, add the broth and the water and combine. Add the xanthan gum and mix.
⇒ Allow broth mixture to come to boil and then transfer the meat back in and cook covered for 30 minutes.
⇒ Stir frequently scraping the bottom as you stir; after 30 minutes, add the carrots and potatoes and cook for 30 minutes, frequently stirring until it thickens. If you feel the need, you can add more water. Serve warm and enjoy!

Nutrition Facts per Serving:
Calories: 498 kcals, **Carbohydrates:** 5g, **Protein:** 17g, **Fat:** 44g, **Sodium:** 313mg, **Potassium:** 287mg, **Phosphorus:** 177mg

Bacon Cheeseburger Soup

Diabetes-friendly recipe
Preparation Time: 20 minutes
Cooking Time: 40 minutes
Servings: 2

Ingredients:
- 2 slices bacon
- 6 ounces ground beef
- 1 cup beef broth
- 1 cup water
- ½ teaspoon garlic powder
- ½ teaspoon onion powder
- 2 teaspoons brown mustard
- ½ teaspoon black pepper
- ½ teaspoon red pepper flakes
- 1 teaspoon cumin
- 1 teaspoon chili powder
- 1 medium dill pickle, diced
- ½ cup shredded cheddar cheese

Directions:
⇒ Start with cooking the bacon in a non- stick pan until crispy, and then set aside.
⇒ Add ground beef in the bacon fat and cook over medium heat for 5 minutes, until browned on both sides.
⇒ Place beef in a cooking pot, add spices and stir well.
⇒ Add broth, water, dill pickle, cheese and stir until combined.
⇒ Simmer for 20 minutes over low heat, stirring occasionally.
⇒ Serve warm or hot with crispy bacon on top.

Nutrition Facts per Serving:
Calories: 339 kcals, **Carbohydrates:** 3g, **Protein:** 14g, **Fat:** 19g, **Sodium:** 286mg, **Potassium:** 275mg, **Phosphorus:** 181mg

Red Pepper & Brie Soup

Vegetarian-friendly recipe
Preparation Time: 5 minutes
Cooking Time: 45 minutes
Servings: 4

Ingredients:
- 1 teaspoon paprika
- 1 teaspoon cumin
- 1 chopped red onion
- 2 chopped garlic cloves
- ¼ cup crumbled brie
- 2 tablespoon extra-virgin olive oil
- 4 chopped red bell peppers
- 4 cups water

Directions:
⇒ Heat the oil in a cooking pot over medium heat.
⇒ Sauté the onions and peppers for 5 minutes over medium heat.
⇒ Add the garlic cloves, cumin, and paprika and sauté for 3 minutes.
⇒ Add the water and allow boiling before turning the heat down to simmer for 30 minutes.
⇒ Remove from the heat and allow cooling slightly.
⇒ Put the mixture in a food processor and blend until smooth.
⇒ Pour into serving bowls and add the crumbled brie to the top with a little black pepper.
⇒ Enjoy!

Nutrition Facts per Serving:
Calories: 140 kcals, **Protein:** 4g, **Carbs:** 9g, **Fat:** 10 , **Sodium:** 69mg, **Potassium:** 347mg, **Phosphorus:** 64mg

Turkey & Lemon-Grass Soup

Diabetes-friendly recipe
Preparation Time: 5 minutes
Cooking Time: 40 minutes
Servings: 4

Ingredients:
- 1 fresh lime
- ¼ cup fresh basil leaves
- 1 tbsp. cilantro
- 1 cup canned and drained water chestnuts
- 1 tbsp. olive oil
- 1 thumb-size minced ginger piece
- 1 finely chopped green chili
- 4 oz. skinless turkey breasts, cooked and shredded
- 1 minced garlic clove, minced
- ½ finely sliced stick lemongrass
- 1 white onion, chopped
- 3 cups water

Directions:
⇒ Crush the lemongrass, cilantro, chili, 1 tablespoon oil and basil leaves in a blender. Set aside.
⇒ Heat a large non-stick pan/wok with 1 tablespoon olive oil on high heat.
⇒ Sauté the onions, garlic and ginger until soft.
⇒ Add the turkey and sauté for 2 minutes.
⇒ Add the water and stir.

⇒ Next add the water chestnuts, turn down the heat slightly and allow to simmer for 25-30 minutes.
⇒ Add lemongrass sauce and serve hot or warm.

Nutrition Facts per Serving:
Calories: 170 kcal, **Protein:** 8 g, **Carbs:** 22 g, **Fat:** 6 g, **Sodium:** 29 mg, **Potassium:** 335 mg, **Phosphorus:** 101 mg

Paprika Pork Soup

Diabetes-friendly recipe
Preparation Time: 5 minutes
Cooking Time: 35 minutes
Servings: 2

Ingredients:
- 4 oz. sliced pork loin
- 1 onion, diced
- 2 minced garlic cloves
- 1 cup baby spinach
- 3 cups water
- 1 tbsp. extra-virgin olive oil
- 1 tablespoon paprika
- 1 teaspoon black pepper

Directions:
⇒ In a large cooking pot add the oil, chopped onion, and minced garlic.
⇒ Sauté for 5 minutes on low heat.
⇒ Add the pork slices to the onions and cook for 5 minutes or until browned.
⇒ Add paprika and water to the pan. Bring to a boil on high heat.
⇒ Stir in the spinach, reduce heat and simmer for 20 minutes
⇒ Season with pepper to serve.

Nutrition Facts per Serving:
Calories: 90 kcals, **Protein:** 7g, **Carbohydrates:** 5g, **Fat:** 5g, **Sodium:** 26mg, **Potassium:** 242mg, **Phosphorus:** 84mg.

Mediterranean Vegetable Soup

Vegetarian-friendly recipe
Preparation Time: 5 minutes
Cooking Time: 30 minutes
Servings: 4

Ingredients:
- 1 tablespoon extra-virgin olive oil
- 1 tablespoon oregano
- 2 minced garlic cloves
- 1 teaspoon black pepper
- 1 diced zucchini
- 1 cup diced eggplant
- 1 cup low sodium chicken stock
- 2 cups water
- 1 diced red pepper
- 1 diced red onion

Directions:
⇒ Soak the vegetables in warm water prior to use.
⇒ In a large cooking pot add oil, chopped onion, and minced garlic.
⇒ Sauté for 5 minutes over medium heat.
⇒ Add the other vegetables to the onions and sauté for 8 minutes.
⇒ Add stock, water and bring to boil.
⇒ Stir in the herbs, reduce the heat, and simmer for a further 20 minutes.
⇒ Season with pepper to serve.

Nutrition Facts per Serving:
Calories: 70 kcals, **Carbohydrates:** 7g, **Protein:** 2g, **Fat:** 4g, **Sodium:** 44mg, **Potassium:** 321mg, **Phosphorus:** 44mg.

Tofu and Zucchini Soup

Vegetarian-friendly recipe
Preparation Time: 5 minutes
Cooking Time: 20 minutes
Servings: 2

Ingredients:
- 1 tablespoon miso paste
- 1/4 cup soft tofu, cubed
- 1 green onion, chopped
- 1 cup zucchini, diced
- ¼ cup Shiitake mushrooms, sliced
- 1 cup glutamate free vegetable stock
- 2 cups water
- 1/2 tablespoon soy sauce

Directions:
⇒ Take a saucepan, pour the stock and the water into this pan and let it boil on high heat. Reduce heat to medium and let this stock simmer. Add mushrooms and zucchini and cook for almost 10 minutes.
⇒ Take a bowl and mix Soy sauce and miso paste together in this bowl.
⇒ Add this mixture and tofu in stock.
⇒ Simmer for nearly 5 minutes and serve with chopped green onion.

Nutrition Facts per Serving:
Calories: 33 kcals, **Fat:** 1 g, **Protein:** 4g, **Carbohydrates:** 4g, **Sodium:** 449mg, **Potassium:** 171mg, **Phosphorus:** 53mg

Onion Soup

Diabetes-friendly
Preparation Time: 10 minutes
Cooking Time: 35 minutes
Servings: 4

Ingredients:
- ½ cup chopped shiitake mushrooms
- 1 tablespoon grated ginger root
- 1 carrot, chopped
- 3 onions, diced
- ½ celery stalk, sliced
- ¼ tablespoon minced garlic
- 1 tablespoon butter
- 1 tablespoon minced chives
- 3 tablespoons beef bouillon
- 2 tablespoons chicken stock
- 2 cups water

Directions:
- ⇒ In a non-stick cooking pot combine butter, carrot, onions, celery, garlic, mushrooms and ginger.
- ⇒ Sauté for 5 minutes.
- ⇒ Add water, beef bouillon and chicken stock. Cook over high heat and let it boil.
- ⇒ Decrease over medium heat and cover. Simmer for 20 minutes.
- ⇒ Serve delicious soup in small bowls and sprinkle chives over each bowl.

Nutrition Facts per Serving:
Calories: 79 Kcals, **Carbohydrates:** 12g, **Protein:** 2g, **Fat:** 3g, **Sodium:** 67mg, **Potassium:** 285mg, **Phosphorus:** 64mg

Roasted Red Pepper Soup

Diabetes-friendly recipe
Preparation Time: 15 minutes
Cooking Time: 45 minutes
Servings: 4

Ingredients:
- 3 red peppers, roasted and sliced
- 2 cups low-sodium chicken stock
- 1 cup water
- 1 cup onions, thinly sliced
- ½ cup fresh cilantro, minced
- 3 tablespoons lemon juice, freshly squeezed
- 1 tablespoon olive oil
- ½ teaspoon black pepper

Directions:
- ⇒ Combine all the ingredients in a medium stockpot. Bring to a boil over high heat.
- ⇒ Reduce heat. Cover and simmer for 30 minutes until thick. Season with lemon, olive oil and add pepper to taste.
- ⇒ Turn off the heat.
- ⇒ Puree the soup with a hand blender or food processor.
- ⇒ Add the cilantro and turn on the heat to gently reheat the pureed soup.
- ⇒ Serve and enjoy

Nutrition Facts per Serving:
Calories: 78 Kcals, **Carbohydrates:** 10g, **Protein:** 2g, **Fat:** 4g, **Sodium:** 77mg, **Potassium:** 277mg, **Phosphorus:** 36mg,

Chicken Soup

Diabetes-friendly recipe
Preparation Time: 15 minutes
Cooking Time: 1 hour 30 minutes
Servings: 6

Ingredients:
- 1 lb frying chicken, skinned and cut into pieces
- 1 cup low sodium chicken stock
- 2 cups water
- 1 cups carrot diced
- 1 cup zucchini diced1 cup onion diced
- 2 teaspoons herb seasoning (see recipe)
- 2 bay leaves
- Lemon and pepper (to taste)

Directions:
- ⇒ Place chicken, bay leaves, chicken stock, water in a large deep cooking pot.
- ⇒ Bring to boil and then reduce heat.
- ⇒ Simmer for 1 hour.
- ⇒ Remove chicken from the pot, shred it chicken and add it back to the pot.
- ⇒ Add mixed vegetables and simmer for 30 minutes.
- ⇒ Season with lemon and add pepper to taste and serve.

Nutrition Facts per Serving:
Calories: 290 Kcals, **Carbohydrates:** 9g, **Protein:** 24g, **Fat:** 18g, **Sodium:** 125mg, **Potassium:** 516mg, **Phosphorus:** 219mg,

Chicken and Rice Soup

Gluten free recipe
Preparation Time: 15 minutes
Cooking Time: 40 minutes
Servings: 4

Ingredients:
- 1 boneless chicken breast, cooked and shredded
- 2 cups low-sodium chicken stock
- 4 cups water
- 3 cups mixed vegetables
- ¾ cup uncooked white rice
- 2 teaspoons lemon pepper or herb seasoning (see recipe)

Directions:
⇒ Combine vegetables, chicken and water in a deep cooking pot.
⇒ Bring to a boil over medium-high heat.
⇒ Cover and reduce heat to simmer for 20 minutes.
⇒ Add chicken stock and rice. Continue simmering 20 more minutes.
⇒ Serve with lemon pepper seasoning or herb seasoning to taste.

Nutrition Facts per Serving:
Calories: 270 Kcals, **Carbohydrates:** 33g, **Protein:** 17g, **Fat:** 6g, **Sodium:** 149mg. **Potassium** 182mg, **Phosphorus:** 139mg,

Pan-Fried White Fish Soup

Diabetes-friendly recipe
Preparation Time: 10 minutes
Cooking Time: 25 minutes
Servings: 4

Ingredients:
- 2 tablespoons olive oil
- 1 lb white fish, cubed
- 1 cup low-sodium vegetable stock
- ½ cup chopped onions
- 3 cups mixed vegetables
- ½ cup fresh chives, chopped
- 2 teaspoons herbal seasoning (see recipe)

Directions:
⇒ Sauté fish with olive oil in a large deep cooking pot for 3 minutes.
⇒ Add the seasoning, stock, and mixed vegetables.
⇒ Bring to boil over high heat and reduce to medium-low heat.
⇒ Cover and simmer for 20 minutes.
⇒ Remove from heat and sprinkle with fresh chives.
⇒ Serve and enjoy.

Nutrition Facts per Serving:
Calories: 220 kcals, **Carbohydrates:** 7g, **Protein:** 22 g, **Fat:** 10g, **Sodium:** 114mg, **Potassium:** 475mg, **Phosphorus:** 247mg.

Tomato and Bean Soup

Diabetes-friendly recipe
Preparation Time: 15 minutes
Cooking Time: 40 minutes
Servings: 6

Ingredients:
- 1 cup low-sodium chicken stock
- 1 cup water
- 1 tablespoon herb seasoning (see recipe)
- 1 cup black beans, drained and rinsed
- 3 cups diced tomatoes
- Black pepper, to taste

Directions:
⇒ Combine all the ingredients in a pot. Whisk the mixture to integrate the black beans into the soup.
⇒ Simmer for 30 minutes.
⇒ Season with freshly ground pepper or add black pepper to taste. Serve warm.

Nutrition Facts per Serving:
Calories: 99 Kcals, **Carbohydrates:** 19g, **Protein:** 5g, **Fat:** 1g, **Sodium:** 508mg, **Potassium:** 553mg, **Phosphorus:** 98mg.

Vegetable Soup

Vegetarian-friendly recipe
Diabetes- friendly recipe
Preparation Time: 10 minutes
Cooking Time: 35 minutes
Servings: 4

Ingredients:
- 1 tablespoon olive oil
- 3 cups low-sodium vegetable stock
- 1 cup leeks
- 1 cup cauliflower
- 1 cup carrots
- 1 bay leaf
- 1 garlic clove, minced
- ¼ teaspoon ground cumin

Directions:
⇒ In a deep cooking pan heat the oil over medium-high heat.
⇒ Sauté the garlic and the vegetables for 2 minutes.
⇒ Add the stock, bay leaf, and cumin. Bring to boil and simmer for 30 minutes. Discard the bay leaf and season with lemon pepper seasoning to taste.

⇒ You can serve this delicious soup as it is or blend it with a hand blender or food processor to puree it.

Nutrition Facts per Serving:
Calories: 52 kcals, **Carbohydrates:** 11 g, **Protein:** 2g, **Fat:** 2g, **Sodium:** 117mg, **Potassium:** 224 mg, **Phosphorus:** 32mg,

Carrot and Ginger Soup

Vegetarian-friendly recipe
Diabetes- friendly recipe
Preparation Time: 10 minutes
Cooking Time: 30 minutes
Servings: 4

Ingredients:
- 1 tablespoon olive oil
- 3 cups carrots, chopped
- 2 cloves garlic, minced
- 4 cups low-sodium vegetable stock (see recipe)
- 1 cup chopped onion
- 1 tablespoon minced ginger

Directions:
⇒ Heat the oil in a cooking pot over medium heat. Sauté carrots, onion, and pepper for 5 minutes.
⇒ Add the ginger and garlic and cook for a minute.
⇒ Add the stock and cover. Simmer for 25.
⇒ Turn off the heat and let it cool.
⇒ Puree with a hand blender or food processor.
⇒ Serve and enjoy.

Nutrition Facts per Serving:
Calories: 96 kcals, **Carbohydrates**: 14g, **Protein:** 2g, **Fat:** 4g, **Sodium:** 182mg, **Potassium:** 354mg, **Phosphorus:** 43mg,

Cream of Mushroom Soup

Vegetarian-friendly recipe
Diabetes- friendly recipe
Preparation Time: 15 minutes
Cooking Time: 30 minutes
Servings: 2

Ingredients:
- 1 tablespoon butter
- 1 cup mushrooms, finely minced
- 1 cup onion, minced
- 3 tablespoons of all-purpose flour
- 2 cups low-sodium vegetable stock
- 1 cup skimmed milk

Directions:
⇒ Melt the butter on a non-stick cooking pot. Sauté the onion until for 5 minutes.
⇒ Add the mushrooms and cook for at least 5 minutes.
⇒ Sprinkle the flour and cook for 1 minute, stirring continuously.
⇒ Slowly add stock and milk and stir until smooth.
⇒ Bring to a simmer and let it cook for 5 minutes or until thick.
⇒ Season with freshly ground pepper or herb seasoning to taste.

Nutrition facts per serving: Calories: 89 kcals, **Carbohydrates**: 12g, **Protein:** 4g, **Fat:** 3g, **Sodium:** 86mg; **Potassium:** 236mg, **Phosphorus:** 98mg,

Chapter 7. Sauces and Seasoning Mixes

Basil Pesto Sauce

Vegetarian-friendly recipe
Preparation Time: 15 minutes
Cooking Time: 0 minutes
Servings: 4

Ingredients:
- 8 tablespoons olive oil
- 1 garlic clove
- 3 cups fresh basil leaves
- 1 tablespoon pine nuts
- 1 teaspoon Parmesan cheese

Directions:
⇒ Put all of the ingredients into a food processor and blend until smooth.
⇒ Store prepared pesto sauce in a jar or covered container until ready to use. Keep it for up to a week in the refrigerator.
⇒ Serve with pasta, pizza, salads.

Nutrition Facts per Serving:
Calories: 272 kcals, **Carbohydrates:** 1g, **Protein:** 1g, **Fat:** 30g, Sodium: 7mg, **Potassium:** 70 mg, **Phosphorus:** 14mg.

Jalapeño Tomato Salsa

Vegetarian-friendly recipe
Preparation Time: 5 minutes
Cooking Time: 0 minutes
Servings: 4

Ingredients:
- 2 jalapeños, seeded and chopped
- 2 garlic cloves, peeled
- ½ white onion, chopped
- 10 oz tomatoes, quartered
- Juice of ½ lime

Directions:
⇒ Add the jalapeños, garlic, onion, tomatoes, and lime juice into a blender.
⇒ Blend this salsa mixture until it gets chunky.
⇒ Serve fresh.

Nutrition Facts per Serving:
Calories: 23 kcals, **Carbohydrate:** 5g, **Protein:** 1g, **Fat:** 1g, **Sodium:** 5mg, **Potassium:** 215mg **Phosphorous:** 26mg,

Seafood Seasoning

Diabetes-friendly recipe
Preparation Time: 15 minutes
Cooking Time: 0 minutes
Servings: 4

Ingredients:
- 5 teaspoons fennel seeds
- 4 teaspoons dried parsley
- 5 teaspoons dried basil
- 1 teaspoon dried lemon peel

Directions:
⇒ Crush up the fennel seeds and put the rest of the items into a jar, shaking to mix.
⇒ Keep sealed until ready to coat fish or seafood.

Nutrition Facts per Serving:
Calories: 15 kcals, **Carbohydrates:** 3 g, **Protein:** 1 g, **Fat:** 1 g, **Sodium:** 5 mg, **Potassium:** 88 mg, **Phosphorus:** 17 mg.

Pizza Sauce

Diabetes-friendly recipe
Vegetarian friendly recipe
Preparation Time: 15 minutes
Cooking Time: 0 minutes
Servings: 4

Ingredients:
- 1 teaspoon oregano
- 1 cup tomatoes, chopped
- 1 teaspoon parsley flakes
- 6 basil leaves (fresh)
- 6 teaspoon olive oil

Directions:
⇒ Mix all of the ingredients together continuously stirring until the sauce has a nice spreadable consistency.
⇒ This quantity is enough for one large pizza.

Nutrition Facts per Serving:
Calories: 72 kcals, **Carbohydrates:** 2 g, **Protein:** 1 g, **Fat:** 7 g, **Sodium:** 3 mg, **Potassium:** 121 mg, **Phosphorus:** 12 mg.

Chicken and Turkey Seasoning

Diabetes-friendly recipe
Preparation Time: 15 minutes
Cooking Time: 0 minutes
Servings: 6

Ingredients:
- 6 teaspoons sage
- 6 teaspoons thyme
- 1 teaspoons ground pepper
- 2 teaspoons dried marjoram

Directions:
⇒ Mix all spices together and keep in an airtight container. Good for up to one year.

Nutrition Facts per Serving:
Calories: 5 kcals, **Carbohydrates:** 1 g, **Protein:** 1 g, **Fat:** 1 g, **Sodium:** 1 mg, **Potassium:** 19 mg, **Phosphorus:** 3 mg.

Garlicky Sauce

Diabetes-friendly recipe
Vegetarian friendly recipe
Preparation Time: 15 minutes
Cooking Time: 0 minutes
Servings: 4

Ingredients:
- ½ cup lemon juice
- ¼ teaspoon salt
- 1 head garlic
- ¼ cup olive oil

Directions:
⇒ Peel apart the cloves of garlic and clean them.
⇒ Place the garlic, half a tablespoon of lemon juice, and salt in the bottom of a blender.
⇒ Pour the olive oil slowly in a thin stream while blending. The mixture should become thick and white, resembling salad dressing.
⇒ Add the remaining lemon juice and continue to blend.
⇒ Keep in a container for 5 days.

Nutrition Facts per Serving:
Calories: 146 kcals, **Carbohydrates:** 5 g, **Protein:** 1 g, **Fat:** 14 g, **Sodium:** 147 mg, **Potassium:** 69 mg, **Phosphorus:** 17 mg.

Pepper and Lemon Seasoning

Vegetarian-friendly recipe
Preparation Time: 15 minutes
Cooking Time: 0 minutes
Servings: 4

Ingredients:
- 1 teaspoons ground coriander seeds
- 2 lemons
- 2 tablespoons cracked peppercorns

Directions:
⇒ Heat an oven to the lowest temperature setting. Wash and dry the lemons. Remove the yellow part of the lemon peel by finely grating it.
⇒ Mix the finely grated lemon zest with the cracked peppercorns.
⇒ Layout the mixture on a flat cooking sheet that has been lined. Put the flat cooking sheet in the oven for one hour and fifteen minutes, stirring mixture for a minimum of every twenty minutes.
⇒ Add the coriander to the mixture and place it all into a food processor to finely grind.
⇒ Store it in an airtight container. It can be used to replace table salt.

Nutrition Facts per Serving:
Calories: 21 kcals, **Carbohydrates:** 6 g, **Protein:** 1 g, **Fat:** 1 g, **Sodium:** 2 mg, **Potassium:** 103 mg, **Phosphorus:** 13 mg

Edamame Guacamole

Vegetarian-friendly recipe
Preparation Time: 10 minutes
Cooking Time: 0 minutes
Servings: 4

Ingredients:
- 1 cup frozen shelled edamame, thawed
- ¼ cup water
- 1 lemon, juice and zest
- 2 tablespoons chopped fresh cilantro
- 1 tablespoon olive oil
- 1 teaspoon minced garlic

Directions:
⇒ In a food processor (or blender), add the edamame, water, lemon juice, lemon zest, cilantro, olive oil, and garlic, and pulse until blended but still a bit chunky.
⇒ Serve fresh.

Nutrition Facts per Serving:
Calories: 63 kcals, **Fat:** 5g, **Carbohydrates:** 12g, **Protein:** 3g, **Sodium:** 3mg, **Phosphorous:** 100mg, **Potassium:** 64mg

Sweet Vinegar Sauce

Vegetarian-friendly recipe
Preparation Time: 15 minutes
Cooking Time: 5 minutes
Servings: 4

Ingredients:
- 4 tablespoons peach jam
- 4 tablespoons brown sugar
- 3 tablespoons apple cider vinegar
- 4 tablespoons butter (unsalted)

Directions:
⇒ Cook everything over low heat in a non-stick frying pan for 5 minutes. Stir the mixture frequently.
⇒ The sauce is best when served hot.

Nutrition Facts per Serving:
Calories: 188 kcals, **Carbohydrates:** 22g, **Protein:** 1g, **Fat:** 11g, **Sodium:** 5 mg, **Potassium:** 25 mg, **Phosphorus:** 5 mg.

BBQ Dry Rub

Diabetes-friendly recipe
Preparation Time: 15 minutes
Cooking Time: 0 minutes
Servings: 4

Ingredients:
- 1 teaspoon chili powder
- 1 teaspoon garlic powder
- 1 teaspoon onion powder
- 3 teaspoons brown sugar
- 1 teaspoon ground cumin
- 1 teaspoon paprika
- ¼ teaspoon dry mustard powder
- ¼ teaspoon. ground red pepper

Directions:
⇒ Add all ingredients to an airtight container and shake to mix thoroughly.
⇒ Rub onto chicken or pork before baking.

Nutrition Facts per Serving:
Calories: 21 kcals, **Carbohydrates:** 5g, **Protein:** 1g, **Fat:** 1g, **Sodium:** 22mg, **Potassium:** 57mg, **Phosphorus:** 13mg.

Cranberry Cabbage

Vegetarian-friendly
Preparation Time: 10 minutes
Cooking Time: 20 minutes
Servings: 4

Ingredients:
- 10 ounces canned whole-berry cranberry sauce
- 1 tablespoon fresh lemon juice
- 1 medium head red cabbage
- 1/4 teaspoon ground cloves

Directions:
⇒ Place the cranberry sauce, lemon juice and cloves in a large cooking pan and bring to a boil.
⇒ Add cabbage and reduce to simmer.
⇒ Cook until the cabbage is tender, stirring occasionally to make sure the sauce does not stick.
⇒ Serve hot with beef, lamb, or pork.

Nutrition Facts per Serving:
Calories: *178 kcals*, **Carbohydrates**: *44g*, **Protein:** *4g*, **Fat:** *19g*, **Sodium:** *61mg*, **Potassium:** *530mg*, **Phosphorus:** *66mg*

Cajun Seasoning

Diabetes-friendly recipe
Preparation Time: 15 minutes
Cooking Time: 0 minutes
Servings: 4

Ingredients:
- 1 teaspoon powdered garlic
- 1 teaspoon ground paprika
- 1 teaspoon powdered onion
- 1 teaspoon medium Cayenne powder

Directions:
⇒ Mix all the ingredients together, put them in a container that is airtight. Spices can be stored for up to 12 months.

Nutrition Facts per Serving:
Calories: 8 kcals, **Carbohydrates:** 2 g, **Protein:** 1g, **Fat:** 1 g, **Sodium:** 2 mg, **Potassium:** 37 mg, **Phosphorus:** 8 mg.

White Alfredo Sauce

Diabetes-friendly recipe
Preparation Time: 15 minutes
Cooking Time: 10 minutes
Servings: 6

Ingredients:
- 6 tablespoons. grated parmesan cheese
- 12 tablespoons skimmed milk
- 1 tablespoon butter
- ½ cup light cream cheese
- ½ teaspoon powdered garlic
- ¼ teaspoon white pepper

Directions:
⇒ Cut up the cheese (cream) in small blocks and put it in a pot.
⇒ Cook on low heat and add in the milk, parmesan cheese, butter, white pepper, and garlic powder.
⇒ Stir until completely melted and well mixed.

Nutrition Facts per Serving:
Calories: 132 kcals, **Carbohydrates:** 5g, **Protein:** 7 g, **Fat:** 9 g, **Sodium:** 217 mg, **Potassium:** 159mg, **Phosphorus:** 145 mg.

Vinaigrette

Vegetarian-friendly recipe
Preparation Time: 15 minutes
Cooking Time: 0 minutes
Servings: 4

Ingredients:
- 1 teaspoon mustard
- 1 teaspoon white wine vinegar
- ½ teaspoon lemon juice
- 3 tablespoons olive oil
- Garlic, crushed, to taste
- Black pepper

Directions:
1. Incorporate mustard, white vinegar, white wine vinegar and lemon juice in a small mixing bowl.
2. Beat in olive oil and add crushed garlic.
3. Blend the mixture and add pepper, if desired.

Nutrition Facts per Serving:
Calories 97 **kcals, Fat:** 0g, **Carbohydrates:** 0g, **Protein:** 0g, **Sodium:** 15 mg, **Phosphorus:** 9 mg, **Potassium:** 3 mg

Healthy Mayonnaise

Vegetarian-friendly recipe
Preparation Time: 5 minutes
Cooking Time: 0 minutes
Servings: 4

Ingredients:
- 1 egg
- ¼ tablespoon Himalayan salt
- 1 teaspoon Dijon mustard
- 2 tablespoons white vinegar
- 2 tablespoons freshly squeezed lemon juice
- 1 cup olive oil
- ½ teaspoon ground pepper

Directions:
⇒ In a mixing bowl, whisk the egg with pepper.
⇒ Whisk in the olive oil until all the oil is used and the mayonnaise is thick and emulsified.
⇒ Add vinegar and lemon juice and stir until completely melted and well mixed.
⇒ Store it in a sealed glass container in the refrigerator for up to 5 days.

Nutrition Facts per Serving:
Calories: 523 kcals, **Carbohydrates:** 1 g, **Protein:** 2 g, **Fat:** 60 g, **Sodium:** 448 mg, **Potassium:** 34 mg, **Phosphorus:** 25 mg,

Tzatziki Sauce

Vegetarian-friendly recipe
Preparation Time: 35 minutes
Cooking Time: 0 minutes
Servings: 4

Ingredients:
- cucumber, grated (2 cups)
- 1 cup 2% plain Greek yogurt
- 1 large clove garlic, minced
- 2 tablespoons extra-virgin olive oil
- 1 tablespoon lemon juice
- 1 tablespoon fresh dill, minced

Directions:
⇒ Place the grated cucumber in a fine-mesh strainer set over a bowl for 10 minutes.
⇒ Use a potato masher and press the cucumber to release the liquid. Repeat two more times for a total of 30 minutes.
⇒ While the cucumber is draining, combine the rest of the ingredients in a mixing bowl.
⇒ Incorporate the cucumber into the mixed ingredients.
⇒ Store refrigerated for up to 3 days.

Nutrition Facts per Serving:
Calories: 74 kcals, **Carbohydrates:** 6g, **Protein:** 3g, **Fat:** 8g, **Sodium:** 40mg, **Potassium:** 208mg, **Phosphorus:** 71mg.

Asian Seasoning

Vegetarian-friendly recipe
Preparation Time: 5 minutes
Cooking Time: 0 minutes
Servings: 6

Ingredients:
- 2 tablespoons sesame seeds
- 2 tablespoons onion powder
- 2 tablespoons crushed star anise pods
- 2 tablespoons ground ginger
- 1 teaspoon ground allspice
- ½ teaspoon cardamom
- ½ teaspoon ground cloves

Directions:
⇒ Mix all the ingredients in a bowl until well incorporated.
⇒ Put the mixture in a jar and store it in a cool and dry place for up to 6 months.

Nutrition Facts per Serving:
Calories: 62 kcals, **Carbohydrates:** 8g, **Protein:** 2g, **Fat:** 4g, **Sodium:** 7 mg
Potassium: 142 mg, **Phosphorus:** 61 mg

Creole Seasoning

Vegetarian-friendly recipe
Preparation Time: 5 minutes
Cooking Time: 0 minutes
Servings: 4

Ingredients:
- 1 tablespoon sweet paprika
- 1 tablespoon garlic powder
- 2 teaspoons onion powder
- 2 teaspoons dried oregano
- 1 teaspoon cayenne pepper
- 1 teaspoon ground thyme
- 1 teaspoon black pepper

Directions:
⇒ Mix all the ingredients in a bowl until well incorporated.
⇒ Put the mixture in a jar and store in a cool and dry place for up to 6 months.

Nutrition Facts per Serving:
Calories: 22 kcals, **Carbohydrates:** 5g, **Protein:** 1g, **Fat:** 1g, **Sodium:** 4 mg, **Potassium:** 107mg, **Phosphorus:** 23 mg.

Yogurt Cream Sauce

Vegetarian-friendly recipe
Preparation Time: 5 minutes
Cooking Time: 10 minutes
Servings: 4

Ingredients:
- 1 medium zucchini, thinly sliced
- 1 teaspoon olive oil
- 2 cloves garlic
- 1 cup pumpkin, sliced
- 1 Bell pepper
- 1 cup low sodium vegetable stock
- ¼ cup fresh basil
- 1 teaspoon Light Cream
- ½ cup Greek yogurt
- ¼ teaspoon salt

Directions:
⇒ Put oil in a large frying pan and heat over medium-high heat. Add zucchini, pumpkin, bell pepper and garlic.
⇒ Reduce heat to low, cook until pepper begins to soften.
⇒ Add stock and simmer for 10 minutes.
⇒ Remove from heat, add yogurt, basil, light cream, salt, and pepper and stir well.
⇒ This sauce is perfect with pasta.

Nutrition Facts per Serving:
Calories: 65 kcals, **Carbohydrates:** 7g, **Protein:** 4g, **Fat:** 3g, **Sodium:** 188 mg, **Potassium:** 336 mg, **Phosphorus:** 77 mg.

Broccoli and Garlic Sauce

Vegetarian-friendly recipe
Preparation Time: 10 minutes
Cooking Time: 15 minutes
Servings: 3

Ingredients:
- 1 cup broccoli floret
- 1 garlic clove
- ½ tablespoon butter
- 1 teaspoon honey
- 1 tablespoon apple cider vinegar
- 1 tablespoon fresh parsley

Directions:
⇒ In a large saucepan with steamer rack, steam broccoli on boiling water 8 to 10 minutes or until crisp-tender (cover with lid while steaming).
⇒ Stir in honey, apple cider vinegar and chopped parsley. Return to the saucepan to heat until sauce is heated.

- ⇒ Add steamed broccoli and blend with a food processor.
- ⇒ Store in the fridge for up to 2 days.

Nutrition Facts per Serving:
Calories: 26 kcals, **Carbohydrates:** 3g, **Protein:** 1g, **Fat:** 2g, **Sodium:** 7 mg, **Potassium:** 68mg, **Phosphorus:** 14 mg

Taco Sauce

Vegetarian-friendly recipe
Preparation Time: 5 minutes
Cooking Time: 15 minutes
Servings: 4

Ingredients:
- o 6 oz tomato sauce (unsalted)
- o 4 tablespoons water
- o 2 teaspoons white vinegar
- o 1 teaspoon ground cumin
- o ¾ teaspoon onion powder
- o ¼ teaspoon garlic powder
- o ¼ teaspoon chili powder
- o ¼ teaspoon paprika
- o ¼ teaspoon white sugar
- o ¼ teaspoon cayenne pepper

Directions:
- ⇒ In a saucepan stir tomato sauce, water, vinegar, cumin, onion powder, garlic salt, chili powder, paprika, sugar, and cayenne pepper.
- ⇒ Simmer over low heat until slightly thickened, about 15 minutes.
- ⇒ Cool sauce slightly before serving.

Nutrition Facts per Serving:
Calories: 17 kcals, **Carbohydrates:** 4g, **Protein:** 1g, **Fat:** 2g, **Sodium:** 11mg, **Potassium:** 153mg, **Phosphorus:** 18mg

Chapter 8. Snacks

Cereal Munch

Gluten-free recipe
Preparation Time: 5 minutes
Cooking Time: 7 minutes
Servings: 3

Ingredients:
- 3 cups cereal, salt-free
- 1 ½ cups oyster crackers, salt-free
- 2 ½ tablespoons butter, unsalted
- ½ cup pretzel twists, salt-free
- ½ tablespoon chili powder
- 1 pinch ground cumin
- ¼ teaspoon garlic powder
- 1 pinch cayenne pepper
- ¾ teaspoons lemon juice

Directions:
⇒ Brush a 10x15 inches pan with melted butter.
⇒ Place the pretzels and crackers with the remaining ingredients in the baking tray and stir gently.
⇒ Bake them for 7 minutes in the oven at 350°F.
⇒ Serve.

Nutrition Facts per Serving:
Calories: 344 kcals, **Carbohydrate:** 53g, **Protein:** 11g, **Fat:** 15g, **Sodium:** 254 mg, **Potassium:** 297 mg, **Phosphorous:** 228 mg

Coconut Mandarin Salad

Vegetarian-friendly recipe
Preparation Time: 5 minutes
Cooking Time: 0 minutes
Servings: 6

Ingredients:
- 14 oz. can pineapple chunks
- 5 oz. canned mandarin oranges
- 5 oz. maraschino cherries, cut in halves
- ½ cup shredded sweetened coconut

Directions:
⇒ Put the pineapples with the cherries, oranges and coconut in a bowl. Serve fresh.

Nutrition Facts per Serving:
Calories: 240 kcals, **Carbohydrate:** 38g, **Protein:** 2g, **Fat:** 10g, **Sodium:** 9mg, **Phosphorous:** 285mg, **Potassium:** 11mg

Cream Dipped Cucumbers

Vegetarian-friendly recipe
Preparation Time: 5 minutes
Cooking Time: 0 minutes
Servings: 4

Ingredients:
- 1/2 cup sour cream
- 3 tablespoons white vinegar
- 1 teaspoon stevia
- Pepper to taste
- 4 cucumbers, peeled and sliced
- 1 small onion, cut into rings

Directions:
⇒ In a medium-sized serving bowl add the liquid ingredients, stevia, pepper and stir well.
⇒ Add cucumber and onion and stir gently.
⇒ Refrigerate for 2 hours.
⇒ Stir again, serve, and enjoy.

Nutrition Facts per Serving:
Calories 89 kcals, **Carbohydrate:** 12g, **Protein:** 2g, **Fat:** 5g, **Sodium:** 16 mg, **Phosphorous:** 370mg, **Potassium:** 78 mg

Puff Pastry Barbecue Cups

Diabetes-friendly recipe
Preparation Time: 15 minutes
Cooking Time: 20 minutes
Servings: 4

Ingredients:
- ½ lb. lean ground turkey
- ¼ cup spicy barbecue sauce
- 2 teaspoons onion flakes
- 1 dash garlic powder
- 8 oz puff pastry

Directions:
⇒ Grease a suitable pan with cooking spray and place it over moderate heat.
⇒ Take a non-stick fry pan to over medium-high heat. Add the ground turkey and sauté it until golden brown.
⇒ With the puff pastry make 8 balls and place them in a muffin tray.

- ⇒ Press each ball in its muffin cup and divide the turkey in it.
- ⇒ Top the turkey with barbecue sauce, garlic powder, and onion flakes.
- ⇒ Bake for 30 minutes at 400°.
- ⇒ Serve and enjoy.

Nutrition Facts per Serving:
Calories: 450 kcals, **Carbohydrates:** 34g, **Protein:** 14g, **Fat:** 29g, **Sodium:** 356mg, **Potassium:** 213mg, **Phosphorus:** 145mg,

Spiced Pretzels

Vegetarian-friendly recipe
Preparation Time: 1 hour 15 minutes
Cooking Time: 10 minutes
Servings: 6

Ingredients:
- ½ teaspoon ground cayenne pepper
- ½ teaspoon lemon pepper
- ½ teaspoon garlic powder
- 1 teaspoon onion powder
- 1 tablespoons corn oil
- 6 oz. unsalted mini pretzels

Directions:
- ⇒ Preheat the oven to 375°F.
- ⇒ Spread the pretzels on a cooking sheet and break them into pieces.
- ⇒ Whisk the oil with the garlic powder, lemon pepper, ground cayenne pepper, and ranch dressing in a bowl.
- ⇒ Pour this oil dressing over the pretzels and toss well to coat.
- ⇒ Bake the pretzels for approximately 5 minutes, then flip them to bake for another 5 minutes.
- ⇒ Serve fresh and warm.

Nutrition Facts per Serving:
Calories: 192 kcals, **Carbohydrates:** 35g, **Protein:** 5g, **Fat:** 4g, **Sodium:** 5 mg, **Potassium:** 94 mg, **Phosphorus:** 18 mg,

Seafood Croquettes

Diabetes-friendly recipe
Preparation Time: 15 minutes
Cooking Time: 10 minutes
Servings: 6

Ingredients:
- 7 oz packed salmon
- 1 egg white
- ¼ cup chopped onion
- ½ teaspoon black pepper
- ½ cup plain breadcrumbs
- 2 tablespoons lemon juice
- ½ teaspoon ground mustard
- ½ teaspoon herb seasoning (see recipe)

Directions:
- ⇒ Drain the packed salmon and transfer it to a bowl.
- ⇒ Stir in all the other ingredients except the oil and mix well.
- ⇒ Make 8 patties out of this mixture and keep them aside.
- ⇒ Add the oil to a non-stick frying pan over medium-high heat.
- ⇒ Add 4 patties at a time and fry them for 3 minutes per side, until golden brown.
- ⇒ Cook the remaining four in the same way.
- ⇒ Serve and enjoy!

Nutrition Facts per Serving:
Calories: 198 kcals, **Carbohydrate:** 19g, **Protein:** 14g, **Fat:** 7g, **Sodium:** 262mg, **Potassium:** 269mg, **Phosphorous:** 150mg

Falafel Balls

Vegetarian-friendly
Preparation Time: 10 minutes
Cooking Time: 10 minutes
Servings: 6

Ingredients:
- 8 oz canned chickpeas, drained and rinsed
- ½ lemon, juiced
- 1 small handful fresh parsley, roughly chopped
- 1 garlic clove, crushed
- ½ teaspoon ground cumin
- ½ teaspoon ground coriander
- 2 tablespoons whole meal flour
- ¼ teaspoon salt
- Black pepper, to taste
- 1 tablespoon olive oil

Directions:
- ⇒ Add chickpeas, lemon juice, parsley, garlic, cumin, coriander, flour, salt and pepper to a food processor. Blend until well combined.
- ⇒ Transfer the mixture into a large bowl. Shape it into 8 falafel balls and flatten slightly between your hands. Cover and refrigerate for 30 minutes.
- ⇒ Heat the oil in a large non-stick frying pan over medium heat. Fry the falafels for 3-4 minutes each side or until golden in color.
- ⇒ Serve hot or warm.

Nutrition Facts per Serving:
Calories: 105 kcals, **Carbohydrate:** 12g, **Protein:** 4g, **Fat:** 5g, **Sodium:** 323mg, **Potassium:** 173mg, **Phosphorous:** 70mg.

Spiced Tortilla Chips

Vegetarian-friendly
Preparation Time: 5 minutes
Cooking Time: 8 minutes
Servings: 4

Ingredients:
- 2(12-inch) flour tortillas, cut into wedges
- ½ teaspoon paprika
- ½ teaspoon rosemary, dried
- ½ teaspoon cayenne pepper
- 2 tablespoons Parmesan cheese

Directions:
⇒ Preheat the oven to 425°F.
⇒ Grease the baking sheet with cooking spray.
⇒ Add all the spices and cheese to a small bowl. Mix well and keep this mixture aside.
⇒ Cut the tortillas into 8 wedges and coat them with the cheese mixture.
⇒ Spread them on a baking tray and drizzle the remaining cheese mixture on top.
⇒ Bake for about 8 minutes at 350°F in a preheated oven.
⇒ Serve hot.

Nutrition Facts per Serving:
Calories: 156 kcals, **Carbohydrate:** 24g, **Protein:** 5g, **Fat:** 5g, **Sodium:** 339mg, **Potassium:** 14mg, **Phosphorous:** 19mg,

Almond Caramel Corn

Vegetarian-friendly recipe
Gluten- free
Preparation Time: 5 minutes
Cooking Time: 5 minutes
Servings: 4

Ingredients:
- 2 ½ cups popped popcorn, unsalted
- 1 cup almonds
- ½ cup brown sugar
- ¼ cup butter
- ¼ cup light corn syrup
- ¼ teaspoon baking soda

Directions:
⇒ Preheat the oven to 425°F.
⇒ Take a shallow roasting pan and spread the almonds and popcorn in it.
⇒ Whisk the brown sugar with the butter and corn syrup in a non-stick saucepan.
⇒ Stir-fry this corn syrup for about 5 minutes up to a boil, then add in the baking soda.
⇒ Pour this corn sauce over the popcorn and almonds in the pan and stir well

⇒ Bake the popcorn mixture for approximately 5 minutes.
⇒ Stir well, then serve.

Nutrition Facts per Serving:
Calories: 494 kcals, **Carbohydrate:** 46g, **Protein:** 9g, **Fat:** 34g, **Sodium:** 62mg, **Potassium:** 369mg, **Phosphorous:** 231mg

Sweet Popped Popcorn

Preparation Time: 5 minutes
Cooking Time: 0 minutes
Servings: 4

Ingredients:
- 4 oz popped popcorn, unsalted
- 2 tablespoons butter
- 2 tablespoons corn syrup
- 2 tablespoons brown sugar
- 1 teaspoon oil

Directions:
⇒ Whisk the corn syrup, brown sugar, and oil in a saucepan.
⇒ Stir-fry the corn syrup mixture for 5 minutes, then remove it from heat.
⇒ Add the butter and mix well, then let the mixture cool. Serve.

Nutrition Facts per Serving:
Calories: 250 kcals, **Carbohydrate:** 29g, **Protein:** 3g, **Fat:** 15g, **Sodium:** 269 mg **Potassium:** 77mg **Phosphorous:** 74 mg,

Cranberry Pecan Salad

Diabetes-friendly recipe
Preparation Time: 5 minutes
Cooking Time: 0 minutes
Servings: 6

Ingredients:
- 1 (12 oz.) package fresh cranberries, chopped
- 1 teaspoon stevia
- 2 cups apples, chopped
- 1/2 cup pecans, chopped
- 1/2 cup low fat vanilla yogurt
- 1 cup frozen whipped topping

Directions:
1. Add the cranberries, apples, stevia, vanilla, pecans to a salad bowl.
2. Add yogurt and topping and stir gently.
3. Refrigerate for 1 hour, then serve.

Nutrition Facts per Serving:
Calories: 236 kcals, **Carbohydrate:** 29g, **Protein:** 3g, **Fat:** 13g, **Sodium:** 22mg, **Potassium:** 245mg, **Phosphorous:** 94mg,

Carrot Corn Bread

Vegetarian-friendly recipe
Preparation Time: 5 minutes
Cooking Time: 30 minutes
Servings: 4

Ingredients:
- 1 cup unbleached flour
- 2 teaspoons baking powder
- 1 egg
- 1 cup skimmed milk
- 2 tablespoons pure maple syrup
- ½ cup sunflower oil
- ½ teaspoon pure vanilla extract
- 1 cup carrot, shredded

Directions:
⇒ Preheat the oven to 400°F.
⇒ Mix the flour with baking powder, egg, milk, maple syrup, sunflower oil, and vanilla extract in a mixer.
⇒ Mix well until smooth, then fold in the carrots.
⇒ Stir well and evenly, then spread the batter in an 8-inch baking pan greased with cooking spray.
⇒ Bake the batter for 30 minutes until golden brown.
⇒ Slice and serve fresh.

Nutrition Facts per Serving:
Calories: 449 kcals, **Carbohydrate:** 40g, **Protein:** 7g, **Fat:** 29g, **Sodium:** 310 mg, **Potassium:** 266mg, **Phosphorous:** 143mg.

Spiced Tortilla Chips

Vegetarian-friendly
Preparation Time: 5 minutes
Cooking Time: 8 minutes
Servings: 6

Ingredients:
- 2 (12-inch) flour tortillas, cut into wedges
- 4 tablespoons olive oil
- ½ teaspoon paprika
- ½ teaspoon rosemary seasoning
- ½ teaspoon cayenne pepper
- Parmesan cheese

Directions:
1. Preheat the oven to 400°F.
2. Grease the baking sheet with cooking spray.
3. Add all the spices and cheese to a small bowl. Mix well and keep this mixture aside.
4. Cut the tortillas into 8 wedges and coat them with the cheese mixture.
5. Spread them on a baking tray and bake for about 8 minutes.
6. Serve fresh.

Nutrition Facts per Serving:
Calories: 156 kcals, **Carbohydrate:** 24g, **Protein:** 5g, **Fat:** 5g, **Sodium:** 339mg, **Potassium:** 14mg, **Phosphorous:** 19mg.

Tuna Dip

Preparation Time: 5 minutes
Cooking Time: 0 minutes
Servings: 6

Ingredients:
- 10 oz canned tuna chunks, drained
- 6 oz Greek yogurt
- ½ teaspoon ground pepper
- ½ cup celery, finely chopped
- 8 rice crackers

Directions:
⇒ Add tuna, celery, yogurt and pepper to a salad bowl.
⇒ Stir them well and refrigerate for 1 hour.
⇒ Serve with rice crackers.

Nutrition Facts per Serving:
Calories: 149 kcals, **Carbohydrate:** 5g, **Protein:** 21g, **Fat:** 4g, **Sodium:** 301 mg, **Potassium:** 276mg, **Phosphorous:** 227mg.

Chicken Bacon Wraps

Diabetes-friendly recipe
Preparation Time: 5 minutes
Cooking Time: 20 minutes
Servings: 4

Ingredients:
- ½ lb chicken breast, 4 thin slices
- 2 thin bacon slices
- ½ teaspoon paprika
- 1 teaspoon garlic, minced
- ¼ teaspoon onion powder
- ½ teaspoon black pepper
- 1 tablespoon olive oil

Directions:
⇒ Preheat the oven to 350°F.
⇒ Wrap each chicken breast with ½ bacon slice and place them in a baking pan.
⇒ Whisk the spices and drizzle over the wrapped chicken.
⇒ Spray the chicken with olive oil.
⇒ Bake for 15 minutes at 350°F.
⇒ Slice and serve.

Nutrition Facts per Serving:
Calories: 187 kcals, **Carbohydrate:** 1g, **Protein:** 15g, **Fat:** 14g, **Sodium:** 220 mg, **Potassium:** 136 mg, **Phosphorous:** 101 mg,

Chapter 9. Salads

Pineapple Cabbage Coleslaw

Vegetarian-friendly recipe
Preparation Time: 15 minutes
Cooking Time: 0 minutes
Servings: 4

Ingredients:
- 12 oz. broccoli coleslaw
- 12 oz. Napa cabbage, finely shredded
- 12 oz. unsweetened pineapple, drained
- 1/2 cup green onions, sliced
- 1 cup Greek yogurt
- 1 tablespoon seasoned rice vinegar
- 1 teaspoon coarse ground black pepper

Directions:
⇒ Cut the pineapple into small pieces and put it in a salad bowl with cabbage and broccoli.
⇒ In a separate small bowl mix yogurt and spices, then drizzle over the veg.
⇒ Refrigerate this coleslaw for at least 1 hour.

Nutrition Facts per Serving:
Calories: 162 kcals, **Carbohydrate:** 29g, **Protein:** 8g, **Fat:** 3g, **Potassium:** 400mg, **Phosphorous:** 104mg,

Lemon peppers salad

Vegetarian-friendly recipe
Preparation Time: 15 minutes
Cooking Time: 0 minutes
Servings: 4

Ingredients:
- 1 cup red pepper, cut into small pieces
- 1 cup yellow pepper, cut into small pieces
- 1 cup green pepper, cut into small pieces
- 2 teaspoons olive oil
- 2 teaspoons lemon juice
- ½ teaspoon black pepper
- 1 teaspoon garlic, minced

Directions:
⇒ In a large serving bowl add green, yellow and red pepper.
⇒ In a separate small bowl add lemon juice, oil, black pepper, garlic and stir well the mixture.
⇒ Pour the dressing mixture in the salad bowl and stir gently.

Nutrition Facts per Serving:
Calories: 45 kcals, **Carbohydrate:** 6g **Protein:** 1g, **Fat:** 3g, **Sodium:** 7mg, **Potassium:** 184mg, **Phosphorous:** 21mg,

Healthy Italian Pinzimonio

Vegetarian-friendly recipe
Preparation Time: 15 minutes
Cooking Time: 0 minutes
Servings: 4

Ingredients:
- 4 celery stalks, halved length-wise
- 2 carrots, cut length-wise in 4 slices
- 2 radishes, halved
- 3 tablespoons olive oil
- 6 tablespoons lemon juice, freshly squeezed
- ½ teaspoon black pepper

Directions:
⇒ Place the vegetables in a shallow serving plate.
⇒ In a small glass bowl add olive oil, lemon juice, black pepper and stir well.
⇒ Put the glass bowl in the center of the serving plate.
⇒ Dip the vegetables in the dressing and enjoy

Nutrition Facts per Serving:
Calories: 127 kcals, **Carbohydrates:** 8g, **Protein:** 1g, **Fat:** 11g, **Sodium:** 57mg, **Potassium:** 303mg, **Phosphorus:** 31mg

Sweet Rice Salad

Gluten-free recipe
Vegetarian- friendly recipe
Preparation Time: 5 minutes
Cooking Time: 0 minutes
Servings: 6

Ingredients:
- 1 tablespoon water
- 1 tablespoon lemon juice

- 2 cups rice, cooked & rinsed
- 1 oz. onion, finely chopped
- 2 apples, chopped
- 8 cherry tomatoes

Directions:
⇒ Mix the rice with the apples, tomatoes, and onion in a salad bowl.
⇒ Whisk the apricot jam and the other dressing ingredients in a small bowl.
⇒ Pour this dressing into the rice salad and mix well.
⇒ Serve.

Nutrition Facts per Serving:
Calories: 440 kcals, **Carbohydrates**: 98g, **Protein:** 8g, **Fat:** 1g, **Sodium:** 7mg, **Potassium:** 298mg, **Phosphorus**: 142mg

Blue Cheese Pear Salad

Diabetes-friendly recipe
Preparation Time: 5 minutes
Cooking Time: 0 minutes
Servings: 6

Ingredients:
- 1 head of lettuce
- ½ red onion, chopped
- 2 pears, peeled, cored and chopped
- ¼ cup pecans, toasted and chopped
- ½ cup blue cheese, crumbled
- 2 tablespoons honey
- ¼ cup apple cider vinegar
- ¼ teaspoon black pepper
- 2 tablespoons olive oil

Directions:
⇒ In a large serving bowl add lettuce, pear, onion.
⇒ In a separate small bowl add honey, cider vinegar, oil, pepper and stir well the mixture.
⇒ Pour the dressing mixture in the salad bowl and stir gently.
⇒ Coat the salad with blue cheese and pecans.
⇒ Serve.

Nutrition Facts per Serving:
Calories: 183 kcals, **Carbohydrate:** 18g **Protein:** 4g, **Fat:** 11g, **Sodium:** 148mg, **Potassium:** 273 mg, **Phosphorous:** 87mg,

Fresh salad

Diabetes-friendly recipe
Preparation Time: 5 minutes
Cooking Time: 0 minutes
Servings: 6

Ingredients:
- 1 head lettuce, sliced
- 4 radishes, sliced
- 2 tablespoons lemon juice, freshly squeezed
- 2 tablespoons olive oil
- ¼ tablespoon black pepper
- ½ tablespoons poppy seeds

Directions:
⇒ In a large serving bowl add lettuce, and radishes.
⇒ In a separate small bowl add lemon juice, oil, pepper and stir well the mixture.
⇒ Pour the dressing mixture in the salad bowl and stir gently.
⇒ Coat the salad with poppy seeds and serve

Nutrition Facts per Serving:
Calories: 54 kcals, **Carbohydrate:** 4g **Protein:** 2g, **Fat:** 4g, **Sodium:** 30mg, **Potassium:** 215mg, **Phosphorous:** 38mg,

Chapter 10. Meat and Poultry Mains

Chicken in Herb Sauce

Preparation Time: 10 minutes
Cooking Time: 33 minutes
Servings: 2

Ingredients:
- 2 skinless chicken breasts
- ½ teaspoon garlic powder
- ¼ teaspoon celery salt
- ¼ teaspoon ground black pepper
- ½ teaspoon paprika
- ¼ teaspoon celery seeds
- ½ teaspoon mustard powder
- 3 tablespoons lemon juice
- 2 tablespoons butter, unsalted
- 1 tablespoon parmesan cheese, grated

Directions:
⇒ Preheat the oven to 350°F.
⇒ Take a small saucepan, place it over medium heat, add butter and when it melts, and add all the ingredients (except for chicken and cheese), stir until mixed, and cook the sauce for 1 minute until hot.
⇒ Remove pan from heat, and then stir in cheese until it melts.
⇒ Take a baking dish, place chicken breasts in it, toss to coat with prepared sauce, and then bake for 30 minutes until the chicken is thoroughly cooked.
⇒ Serve hot.

Nutrition Facts per Serving:
Calories: 230 kcals, **Carbohydrates:** 2g, **Protein:** 32g, **Fat:** 10g **Sodium:** 169mg, **Potassium:** 502 mg, **Phosphorus:** 317mg.

Chicken with Garlic Sauce

Diabetes-friendly recipe
Preparation Time: 10 minutes
Cooking Time: 30 minutes
Servings: 6

Ingredients:
- 2 skinless chicken breasts
- 1 tablespoon garlic, minced
- ½ teaspoon ground black pepper
- 1 tablespoon rosemary leaves, chopped
- ½ cup balsamic vinegar
- 2 tablespoons olive oil
- ½ cup white wine
- 2 cups chicken broth, low-sodium

Directions:
⇒ Take a 9-by-13 inches baking dish, add rosemary, wine, and vinegar, pour in the broth, stir until mixed, add chicken, and let it marinate for a minimum of 4 hours.
⇒ Then take a large non-stick frying pan, place it over medium-high heat, add oil and when hot, add sliced garlic and cook for 2 minutes, or until golden.
⇒ Add marinated chicken, sprinkle with black pepper, and cook for 1 minute per side until golden.
⇒ Then switch over medium heat, pour marinade over the chicken, add garlic and simmer the chicken for 15 minutes until cooked, turning halfway.
⇒ When done, transfer chicken to a dish, switch to high heat, and bring the sauce to a boil, then switch heat to medium-high and simmer the liquid until thickened.
⇒ Drizzle liquid over chicken and then serve.

Nutrition Facts per Serving:
Calories: 297 kcals, **Carbohydrates:** 8g, **Protein:** 34g, **Fat:** 11g, **Sodium:** 361mg, **Potassium:** 636mg, **Phosphorus:** 334mg.

Chicken with Mushroom Sauce

Preparation Time: 10 minutes
Cooking Time: 55 minutes
Servings: 4

Ingredients:
- 1 lb skinless chicken breast
- 1 cup mushrooms, sliced
- 2 bulbs of garlic
- 2 teaspoon herb seasoning
- ½ teaspoon dried thyme
- ¼ teaspoon ground black pepper
- ½ cup all-purpose white flour
- 4 teaspoons olive oil
- ½ cup skimmed milk
- 1 ½ cups chicken broth, low sodium

Directions:

⇒ Preheat the oven to 350°F.
⇒ Cut the top from each bulb of garlic, place bulb on a large piece of foil, cut-side up, drizzle with oil, wrap bulbs tightly, and then bake for 45 minutes, or until tender.
⇒ Meanwhile, wrap each chicken breast in a plastic wrap, and then pound with a meat mallet until ¼-inch thick.
⇒ Place flour in a shallow dish, stir in salt, thyme, and black pepper until combined, reserve 3 tablespoons of this mixture, and use the remaining mixture to coat the chicken.
⇒ Then take a large non-stick frying pan over medium-high heat, add 2 tablespoons olive oil and chicken; cook for 8 minutes. When done, transfer chicken to a plate, cover with foil to keep it warm, and set aside until needed.
⇒ When the garlic has baked, cool garlic bulbs for 10 minutes, then gently squeeze the cloves, chop the garlic, and set aside until required.
⇒ Add remaining oil in a skillet pan with mushrooms and cook for 5 minutes, or until golden brown.
⇒ Sprinkle the reserved flour mixture over mushrooms, stir, cook for 2 minutes, add garlic, pour in milk and broth, stir until well combined, and bring the mixture to a boil.
⇒ Switch to low heat, simmer the mushroom sauce for 3 minutes until the sauce has thickened slightly, add chicken and coat it with the sauce. Cook for 2 more minutes.
⇒ Serve straight away.

Nutrition Facts per Serving:
Calories: 287 kcals, **Carbohydrates:** 21g, **Protein:** 31g, **Fat:** 8g, **Sodium:** 477mg, **Potassium:** 679mg, **Phosphorus:** 355mg,

Beef chorizo

Diabetes-friendly recipe
Preparation time: 10 minutes
Cooking time: 10 minutes
Servings: 4

Ingredients:
o 3 garlic cloves, minced
o 1 lb. 90% lean ground beef
o 2 tbsp. hot chili powder
o 2 tsp. red or cayenne pepper
o 1 tsp. black pepper
o 1 tsp. ground oregano
o 2 tsp. white vinegar

Directions:
⇒ Mix all ingredients together in a bowl thoroughly then spread the mixture in a baking pan.

⇒ Bake the meat for 10 minutes at 325°F in the oven.
⇒ Slice and serve in crumbles.

Nutrition Facts per Serving:
Calories: 72 kcals, **Protein:** 8g, **Carbohydrates:** 1g, **Fat:** 4g, **Sodium:** 46 mg, **Potassium:** 174 mg, **Phosphorus:** 79 mg

Basil Lemon Turkey

Diabetes-friendly recipe
Preparation Time: 10 minutes
Cooking Time: 25 minutes
Servings: 4

Ingredients:
o 1 pound turkey breast, sliced
o 4 teaspoons unsalted butter
o 1 cup water
o 1/4 cup fresh basil, minced
o 1/4 teaspoon garlic powder
o 1/4 teaspoon oregano
o 2 tablespoons lemon zest, grated

Directions:
⇒ Preheat oven to 325°F.
⇒ In a small ball combine basil, garlic, oregano and lemon zest.
⇒ Place the sliced breast in a roasting pan and add a cup of hot water.
⇒ Pour spice mixture evenly over turkey breasts making sure it is smoothly distributed. Pierce the turkey with a fork several times to allow the mixture to season and flavor as it cooks.
⇒ Add 1 teaspoon of butter on top of each slice.
⇒ Bake uncovered, for 25 minutes or until juices in the turkey are clear, not pink.

Nutrition Facts per Serving:
Calories: 167 kcals, **Carbohydrates:** 1g, **Protein:** 27g, **Fat:** 5g, **Sodium:** 129mg, **Potassium:** 323mg, **Phosphorus:** 237mg

Lamb with Prunes

Preparation Time: 15 minutes
Cooking Time: 1 hour 40 minutes
Serving: 4

Ingredients:
o 2 tablespoons coconut oil
o 1 onion, chopped finely
o ½ piece fresh ginger, minced

- 1 garlic clove, minced
- ½ teaspoon ground turmeric
- 1 pound lamb shoulder, trimmed and cubed into 2-inch size
- ground black pepper, to taste
- ¼ teaspoon saffron threads, crumbled
- ½ cinnamon stick
- 2 cups water
- ½ cup prunes, pitted and halved

Directions:
⇒ In a big saucepan, melt coconut oil on medium heat.
⇒ Add onions, ginger, garlic cloves, and turmeric and sauté for about 3 minutes.
⇒ Sprinkle the lamb with black pepper evenly.
⇒ In the pan, add lamb and saffron threads and cook for approximately 4–5 minutes.
⇒ Add cinnamon stick and water and boil on high heat.
⇒ Reduce the temperature to low and simmer, covered for around 1 hour or till the desired doneness of lamb.
⇒ Stir in prunes and simmer for approximately 20 minutes.
⇒ Remove cinnamon stick and serve hot.

Nutrition Facts per Serving:
Calories: 393 kcals, **Carbohydrates:** 17g, **Protein:** 20g, **Fat:** 31g, **Sodium:** 74mg, **Potassium:** 480mg, **Phosphorus:** 205mg

Cabbage Rolls with Chicken

Vegetarian-friendly recipe
Preparation Time: 15 minutes
Cooking Time: 30 minutes
Servings: 4

Ingredients:
- 8 cabbage leaves
- 1 pound ground chicken
- 1/2 cup cooked white rice
- 1/4 cup onion, finely chopped
- 2 egg whites
- 1/2 teaspoon black pepper (divided use)
- 1/4 teaspoon dried basil
- 1–1/4 cup water (divided use)
- 2 tablespoons lemon juice
- 1 tablespoon honey

Directions:
⇒ Preheat the oven to 375°F.
⇒ Carefully remove cabbage leaves from a whole cabbage and wash them.
⇒ Boil a large pot of water. Add cabbage leaves and cook for 2 minutes to soften. Drain and set leaves aside.
⇒ In a large bowl, combine ground chicken, rice, onion, egg whites, 1/4 teaspoon pepper, basil and 1/4 cup water.
⇒ Place 1/4 cup of the chicken mixture on each cabbage leaf and fold sides of the leaf over the chicken mixture.
⇒ Place rolls close together, seam side down in a baking dish.
⇒ Combine lemon juice, 1 cup water, 1/4 teaspoon pepper, and honey to make a sauce. Top cabbage rolls with sauce. Cover and bake at 375°F for 1-1/2 hour. Uncover and bake 30 minutes longer.
⇒ Serve warm and enjoy.

Nutrition Facts per Serving:
Calories: 288 kcals, **Carbohydrates:** 27g, **Protein:** 24g, **Fat:** 14g, **Sodium:** 151mg, **Potassium:** 225mg, **Phosphorus:** 222mg

Turkey and Apple Curry

Diabetic-friendly recipe
Preparation Time: 15 minutes
Cooking Time: 50 minutes
Servings: 4

Ingredients:
- 1 pound skinless boneless turkey breast, sliced
- ¼ teaspoon black pepper
- 1 medium apple, peeled, cored, and finely chopped
- 1 small onion, chopped
- 1 garlic clove, minced
- 1 tablespoons olive oil
- 1 tablespoon curry powder
- ½ tablespoon dried basil
- 1 tablespoon all-purpose flour
- ½ cup low-Sodium chicken broth
- ½ cup soy milk

Directions:
⇒ Preheat oven to 350°F.
⇒ Arrange turkey breast slices in a single layer in a 9 x 13-inch (or larger) baking dish, adding pepper to taste. Set aside.
⇒ In a saucepan, sauté apple, onion, and garlic in olive oil over medium heat until tender.
⇒ Add curry powder and basil; mix well, and sauté for another minute.
⇒ Stir in the flour and continue to cook one minute longer.
⇒ Add chicken broth and soy milk, stirring well. Remove from heat.
⇒ Pour sauce mixture over turkey breasts and bake for 40 minutes.
⇒ Serve hot and enjoy.

Nutrition Facts per Serving:
Calories: 225 kcals, **Carbohydrates:** 13g, **Protein** 29g, **Fat:** 6g, **Sodium:** 254mg, **Potassium:** 453mg, **Phosphorus:** 260mg

Beef and Three Pepper Stew

Diabetes-friendly recipe
Preparation Time: 15 minutes
Cooking Time: 2 hours and 45 minutes
Servings: 6

Ingredients:
- 12 ounces flat-cut beef brisket, whole
- 1 teaspoon dried thyme
- 1 teaspoon black pepper
- 1 garlic clove
- ½ cup green onion, thinly sliced
- 2 ½ cups water
- 1 tablespoon herb seasoning (see recipe)
- 1 large green bell pepper, sliced
- 1 large red bell pepper, sliced
- 1 large yellow bell pepper, sliced
- 1 large red onion, sliced

Directions:
⇒ In a large saucepan put beef, spices and water and sauté over medium heat.
⇒ Switch to low heat and for 2 hours, stirring every 20 minutes.
⇒ Add the sliced peppers and the onion.
⇒ Cook this over medium heat for 25 minutes, until the vegetables are tender.
⇒ Serve hot and enjoy.

Nutrition Facts per Serving:
Calories: 252 kcals, **Carbohydrate:** 9g, **Protein:** 17g, **Fat:** 17g, **Sodium:** 130 mg, **Potassium:** 520mg, **Phosphorous:** 188mg.

Sticky Pulled Beef Open Sandwiches

Preparation Time: 15 minutes
Cooking Time: 2 hours
Servings: 4

Ingredients:
- ½ cup green onion, sliced
- 1 garlic clove, minced
- 1 large carrot, grated
- 7 ounce flat-cut beef brisket, whole
- 1 tablespoon smoked paprika
- 1 teaspoon brown sugar
- ½ teaspoon black pepper
- 2 tablespoon olive oil
- ¼ cup red wine
- 6 tablespoon cider vinegar
- 3 cups water
- 4 thick slices white bread
- ½ cup arugula to garnish

Directions:
⇒ Finely chop the green onion and the garlic. Grate the carrot.
⇒ Put the beef in a non-stick cooking pot.
⇒ Add the chopped onion, garlic, grated carrot and remaining ingredients, leaving the rolls and arugula to one side.
⇒ Stir in to combine all the ingredients except arugula.
⇒ Cover and cook at low heat for 2 hours.
⇒ Remove the meat from the pot and shred it apart with two forks.
⇒ Return the meat to the broth to keep it warm until ready to serve.
⇒ Lightly toast the bread and top with shredded beef, arugula, and ½ spoon of the broth.

Nutrition Facts per Serving:
Calories: 306 kcals, **Carbohydrate:** 20g, **Protein:** 13g, **Fat:** 18g, **Sodium:** 208 mg, **Potassium:** 370 mg, **Phosphorous:** 143 mg.

Herby Beef Stroganoff and Fluffy Rice

Preparation Time: 15 minutes
Cooking Time: 1 hour and 16 minutes
Servings: 4

Ingredients:
- ½ cup onion
- 2 garlic cloves
- 6 ounces flat-cut beef brisket, cut into 1" cubes
- 1/3 cup red wine
- ½ teaspoon dried oregano
- ¼ teaspoon freshly ground black pepper
- ½ teaspoon dried thyme
- ½ teaspoon of saffron
- 2 ½ cups of water
- 1 cup of white rice

Directions:
⇒ Chop up the onion and mince the garlic cloves.
⇒ In a large non-stick pot put onion, garlic, beef, wine, pepper, oregano and thyme.
⇒ Cover and cook at low heat for 1 hour.
⇒ Add rice and water to the pot and stir well. Cook for 10 minutes.
⇒ Add the saffron and simmer for other 6 minutes, stirring continuously with a wooden spoon, until the water is completely absorbed.
⇒ Serve hot and enjoy.

Nutrition Facts per Serving:
Calories: 303 kcals, **Carbohydrate:** 37g, **Protein:** 15g, **Fat:** 13g, **Sodium:** 51 mg, **Potassium:** 237mg, **Phosphorous:** 141mg,

Chunky Beef and Potato Slow Roast

Diabetes-friendly recipe
Preparation Time: 15 minutes
Cooking Time: 5–6 hours
Servings: 6

Ingredients:
- 1 cup peeled potatoes, chunked
- ½ cup onions, sliced
- 1 garlic clove, chopped
- 1 lb flat-cut beef brisket, fat trimmed
- 2 cups water
- 1 teaspoon chili powder
- 1 tablespoon dried rosemary
- 1 tablespoon freshly grated horseradish
- 4 tablespoon lemon juice (freshly squeezed)
- 1 teaspoon cayenne pepper
- 1 tablespoon coconut oil
- ½ cup water

Directions:
⇒ Double boil the potatoes to reduce their potassium content.
⇒ Place the beef brisket in a cooking pot.
⇒ Combine water, chopped garlic, onion, chili powder, and rosemary
⇒ Pour the mixture over the brisket.
⇒ Cover and cook over low heat for 2 hours, until the meat is very tender.
⇒ Drain the potatoes and add them to the pot.
⇒ Cook covered over medium heat for 30 minutes, until the potatoes are tender.
⇒ Prepare the horseradish sauce by whisking together horseradish, lemon juice, minced garlic, coconut oil and cayenne pepper.
⇒ Serve warm and enjoy

Nutrition Facts per Serving:
Calories: 363 kcals, **Carbohydrate:** 11g, **Protein:** 22g, **Fat:** 25g **Sodium:** 85mg, **Potassium:** 562mg, **Phosphorous:** 234 mg.

Chicken and Dumplings

Diabetes-friendly recipe
Preparation Time: 5 minutes
Cooking Time: 0 minutes
Servings: 4

Ingredients:
- 1 lb chopped chicken
- 2 cups water
- 1 stalk celery with leaves, cut fine
- 2 carrots, sliced
- ½ teaspoon black pepper
- ½ teaspoon mace or nutmeg
- ½ cup skimmed milk
- baking powder teaspoons
- 1 cup flour
- 2 tablespoons unsalted butter

Directions:
⇒ Put chicken, vegetables, spices, and water or broth into a cooking pan.
⇒ Add more water, enough to cover the chicken by about 1".
⇒ Cook over low heat for 2 hours.
⇒ Remove the chicken to an ovenproof dish. Remove the bones if you want; they may just fall off. Cover and keep warm.
⇒ With a food processor blend the butter and wet ingredients to a stiff dough and drop by spoonful into the boiling broth.
⇒ Cover the pot, reduce the heat to prevent boiling, and cook for 10 minutes without removing the lid.
⇒ Put the chicken in the large serving dish and serve with dumplings.

Nutrition Facts per Serving:
Calories: 433 kcals, **Carbohydrate:** 29g, **Protein:** 26g, **Fat:** 23g, **Sodium:** 248mg, **Potassium:** 428mg, **Phosphorous:** 271mg

Chicken Lasagna with White Sauce

Diabetes-friendly recipe
Preparation Time: 5 minutes
Cooking Time: 30 minutes
Servings: 4

Ingredients:
- 2 cups chicken meat, diced
- 2 cups water
- 2 tablespoons olive oil
- ½ onion, diced
- 1 teaspoon oregano
- ½ teaspoon black pepper
- ½ cup mushrooms, thick sliced
- 2 flour tablespoons
- 1 cup skimmed milk
- 1 teaspoon nutmeg
- 1 cups mozzarella cheese, grated
- 1 cup zucchini, sliced into little moons
- 12 no-boil lasagna noodles

Directions:
⇒ Preheat the oven to 375°F.
⇒ Place chicken, onions and water in a small pot and bring to boil; reduce heat to simmer for 30 minutes.
⇒ Add mushrooms, zucchini, oregano, black pepper and simmer for 20 minutes.

⇒ In a food processor blend flour, olive oil, milk and nutmeg. Cook this mixture in a small cooking pot at low heat for 5 minutes, stirring continuously.

⇒ In the bottom of a 13x9 inch baking dish, spread 1/3 of the chicken and 1/3 of the white sauce. Arrange 4 lasagna noodles over mixture and repeat. Top with remaining 1/3 of chicken, white sauce. Top with grated mozzarella.

⇒ Cover in foil and place in the oven for 30 minutes. Remove foil for the last 10 minutes until desired crispiness.

Nutrition Facts per Serving:
Calories: 483 kcals, **Carbohydrate:** 54g, **Protein:** 29g, **Fat:** 16g, **Sodium:** 246mg, **Potassium:** 430mg, **Phosphorous:** 323mg,

Chicken with Cornbread Stuffing

Preparation Time: 5 minutes
Cooking Time: 1 hour 10 minutes
Servings: 4

Ingredients:
- 4 pieces boneless, skinless chicken breast halves
- 1 tablespoon unsalted butter
- 1 cup celery, chopped
- 1/2 cup onion, chopped
- 1 teaspoon sage
- 1 teaspoon rosemary
- 1 teaspoon thyme
- ½ teaspoon black pepper
- 1 cup unseasoned croutons
- 1 cup fat free low sodium chicken broth

Directions:
⇒ Preheat oven to 350°F.
⇒ Combine all the spices in a small bowl and coat chicken breasts on both sides with seasoning blend mixture.
⇒ Add chicken breasts to a non-stick fry pan, cook 3 minutes on each side.
⇒ Remove chicken breasts from pan, set aside.
⇒ Melt butter in the pan over low heat. Add celery, onion, ½ cup of water and cook over medium heat 7 minutes or until vegetables are tender.
⇒ Remove from heat.
⇒ Combine cornbread crumbs and croutons in a mixing bowl. Add vegetable mixture and broth, mixing to blend.
⇒ Top the chicken with this mixture and bake at 350°F 25 minutes.
⇒ Remove cover; continue baking 10 minutes.

⇒ Garnish with fresh celery leaves, if desired.

Nutrition Facts per Serving:
Calories: 310 kcals, **Carbohydrate:** 9g, **Protein:** 46g, **Fat:** 8.3g, **Sodium:** 300 mg, **Potassium:** 779mg, **Phosphorous:** 446mg,

Spiced Lamb Burgers

Diabetes-friendly recipe
Preparation Time: 10 minutes
Cooking Time: 20 minutes
Servings: 2

Ingredients:
- 1 tablespoon extra-virgin olive oil
- 1 teaspoon cumin
- ½ red onion, finely diced
- 1 garlic clove, minced
- 1 teaspoon harissa spices
- 1 juiced lemon
- 6-ounce lean ground lamb
- ½ cup low-fat plain yogurt
- 1 head lettuce

Directions:
⇒ Preheat the broiler on medium to high heat.
⇒ Mix together the ground lamb, red onion, Harissa spices until combined.
⇒ Shape 1-inch-thick patties using wet hands.
⇒ Add the patties to a baking tray and place under the broiler for 7–8 minutes on each side or until thoroughly cooked through.
⇒ Mix the yogurt, lemon juice, and cumin, and serve over the lamb burgers with a side salad of fresh lettuce.
⇒

Nutrition Facts per Serving:
Calories: 132 kcals, **Carbohydrate:** 7g, **Protein:** 11g, **Fat:** 7g, **Sodium:** 82mg, **Potassium:** 296mg, **Phosphorous:** 80mg,

Chicken Stuffed Avocado

Diabetes-friendly recipe
Preparation Time: 10 minutes
Cooking Time: 15 minutes
Servings: 4

Ingredients:
- 2 cup grass-fed cooked chicken, shredded
- 2 avocados, halved and pitted
- 1 tablespoon fresh lime juice

- ¼ cup yellow onion, chopped finely
- ¼ cup plain Greek yogurt
- 1 teaspoon Dijon mustard
- Pinch of cayenne pepper
- ½ teaspoon ground black pepper

Directions:
⇒ With a spoon, scoop out the flesh from the middle of each avocado half and transfer it into a bowl.
⇒ Add the lime juice and mash until well combined.
⇒ Add remaining ingredients and stir to combine.
⇒ Divide the chicken mixture into avocado halves evenly and serve immediately.

Nutrition Facts per Serving:
Calories: 273 kcals, **Carbohydrate:** 8g, **Protein:** 14g, **Fat:** 21g, **Sodium:** 56mg, **Potassium:** 526mg, **Phosphorous:** 152mg,

Pork Loins with Leeks

Diabetes-friendly recipe
Preparation Time: 10 minutes
Cooking Time: 35 minutes
Servings: 2

Ingredients:
- 1 sliced leek
- 1 tablespoon mustard seeds
- 8-ounce Pork tenderloin
- 1 tablespoon cumin seeds
- 1 tablespoon dry mustard
- 1 tablespoon extra-virgin oil

Directions:
⇒ Preheat the broiler to medium-high heat.
⇒ In a dry skillet, heat mustard and cumin seeds until they start to pop (3–5 minutes).
⇒ Grind seeds using a pestle and mortar or blender and then mix in the dry mustard.
⇒ Coat the pork on both sides with the mustard blend and add to a baking tray to broil for 25–30 minutes or until cooked through. Turn once halfway through.
⇒ Remove and place to one side.
⇒ Heat the oil in a pan on medium heat and add the leeks for 5–6 minutes or until soft.
⇒ Serve the pork tenderloin on a bed of leeks and enjoy!

Nutrition Facts per Serving:
Calories: 141kcals, **Carbohydrate:** 5g, **Protein:** 13g, **Fat:** 8g, **Sodium:** 37mg, **Potassium:** 323mg, **Phosphorous:** 189mg

Chinese Beef Wraps

Diabetes-friendly recipe
Preparation Time: 10 minutes
Cooking Time: 30 minutes
Servings: 2

Ingredients:
- 4 iceberg lettuce leaves
- 1 diced cucumber
- 1 teaspoon corn oil
- 6-ounce lean ground beef
- 1 teaspoon ground ginger
- 1 tablespoon chili flakes
- 1 garlic clove, minced
- 2 tablespoons rice vinegar

Directions:
⇒ Mix the ground meat with garlic, rice wine vinegar, chili flakes, and ginger in a bowl.
⇒ Heat oil in a fry pan over medium heat.
⇒ Add the beef to the pan and cook for 10 minutes or until cooked through.
⇒ Serve beef mixture with diced cucumber in each lettuce wrap and fold.

Nutrition Facts per Serving:
Calories: 101kcals, **Carbohydrate:** 4g, **Protein:** 9g, **Fat:** 6g, **Sodium:** 31mg, **Potassium:** 260mg, **Phosphorous:** 96mg,

Grilled Skirt Steak

Diabetes-friendly recipe
Preparation Time: 15 minutes
Cooking Time: 8-9 minutes
Servings: 4

Ingredients:
- 2 teaspoons fresh ginger herb, finely grated
- 2 teaspoons fresh lime zest, finely grated
- ¼ cup coconut sugar
- 2 tablespoons fresh lime juice
- ½ cup coconut milk
- 1 lb beef skirt steak, trimmed and cut into 4-inch slices lengthwise
- 1 head lettuce

Directions:
⇒ In a sizable sealable bag, mix together all ingredients except steak.
⇒ Add steak and coat with marinade generously.
⇒ Seal the bag and refrigerate to marinate for about 4 hours.

- ⇒ Preheat the grill to high heat.
- ⇒ Remove steak from refrigerator and discard the marinade.
- ⇒ With a paper towel, dry the steak and cook for approximately 3½ minutes.
- ⇒ Flip the medial side and cook for around 2½-5 minutes or till desired doneness.
- ⇒ With a clear, crisp knife cut into desired slices and serve with fresh lettuce salad.

Nutrition Facts per Serving:
Calories: 352 kcals, **Carbohydrate:** 17g, **Protein:** 24g,
Fat: 22g, **Sodium:** 103mg, **Potassium:** 556mg,
Phosphorous: 221mg,

Spicy Lamb Curry

Diabetes-friendly recipe
Preparation Time: 10 minutes
Cooking Time: 45 minutes
Servings: 6

Ingredients:
- 4 teaspoons ground coriander
- 4 teaspoons ground cumin
- ¾ teaspoon ground ginger
- 2 teaspoons ground cinnamon
- ½ teaspoon ground garlic cloves
- ½ teaspoon ground cardamom
- 2 tablespoons sweet paprika
- ½ tablespoon cayenne pepper
- 2 teaspoons chili powder
- 1-pound boneless lamb, trimmed and cubed into 1-inch size
- ground black pepper, to taste
- 1¼ cups water
- 1 cup coconut milk

Directions:
- ⇒ For spice mixture in a bowl, mix together all spices. Keep aside.
- ⇒ Season the lamb with black pepper.
- ⇒ In a large Dutch oven, heat oil on medium-high heat.
- ⇒ Add lamb and cook for approximately 4–5 minutes.
- ⇒ Stir in the spice mixture and cook for approximately 1 minute.
- ⇒ Add the remaining water and coconut milk and provide to some boil on high heat.
- ⇒ Reduce the heat to low and simmer, covered for approximately 40 minutes or till the desired doneness of lamb.
- ⇒ Serve hot.

Nutrition Facts per Serving:
Calories: 455 kcals, **Carbohydrate:** 11g, **Protein:** 23g,
Fat: 36g, **Sodium:** 168mg,
Potassium: 611mg, **Phosphorous:** 271mg.

Sweet and Sour Chicken

Gluten-free recipe
Preparation Time: 5 minutes
Cooking Time: 40 minutes
Servings: 4

Ingredients:
- 1 can of 12 oz. pineapple
- 2 cornstarch tablespoons
- 1/2 cup vinegar
- 2 orange marmalade tablespoons
- 1/4 cup butter
- 1-pound boneless chicken breast, cut into 1/2-inch cubes
- 1green bell pepper, sliced
- 1 medium onion, thinly sliced and separated into rings
- 1 cup cooked hot white rice (unsalted)

Directions:
- ⇒ Drain the pineapple and store 1/3 cup of the juice.
- ⇒ Combine pineapple juice, cornstarch and vinegar. Put aside.
- ⇒ Melt the butter in a wok or large fry pan.
- ⇒ Add the chicken and cook for 15 minutes, stirring regularly.
- ⇒ Add the green pepper and onion and cook for 15 minutes. Add the pineapple mixture.
- ⇒ Bring to a boil, stirring occasionally.
- ⇒ Serve hot with rice.

Nutrition Facts per Serving:
Calories: 438 kcals, **Carbohydrate:** 35g, **Protein:** 26g,
Fat: 22g, **Sodium:** 181mg, **Potassium:** 464 mg,
Phosphorous: 234 mg.

Roast Beef

Diabetes-friendly recipe
Preparation Time: 25 minutes
Cooking Time: 55 minutes
Servings: 6

Ingredients:
- 2-pounds quality rump or sirloin tip roast
- 1 teaspoon dried rosemary
- 1teaspoon garlic, minced
- 1 teaspoon dried thyme
- 1 teaspoon black pepper
- 2 teaspoons olive oil

- o   1 head lettuce
- o   1 carrot, grated

Direction:
⇒ Preheat the oven to 400°F
⇒ Brush olive oil onto meat, season with pepper and herbs and moist.
⇒ Place the beef on a roasting tray, then place it in the oven.
⇒ Cook for 1 hour for medium beef. If you prefer it medium-rare, take it out 5 to 10 minutes earlier. For well done, leave it in for 10 to 15 minutes longer.
⇒ When the beef is cooked, remove it from the oven and transfer it to a board to rest for about 15 minutes.
⇒ With a very sharp knife cut into thin slices.
⇒ Serve warm or cool with fresh lettuce and grated carrots side salad.

Nutrition Facts per Serving:
Calories: 250 kcals, **Carbohydrate:** 4g, **Protein:** 34g, **Fat:** 12g, **Sodium:** 101mg, **Potassium:** 674mg, **Phosphorous:** 309mg.

Beef Brochettes

Diabetes-friendly recipe
Preparation Time: 20 minutes
Cooking Time: 20 minutes
Servings: 2

Ingredients:
- o   1 ½ cups pineapple chunks
- o   1 sliced large onion
- o   2 pounds thick steak
- o   1 sliced medium bell pepper
- o   1 bay leaf
- o   ¼ cup olive oil
- o   ½ cup lemon juice
- o   2 crushed garlic cloves

Directions:
⇒ Cut beef cubes and place in a plastic bag
⇒ Combine marinade ingredients in small bowl
⇒ Mix and pour over beef cubes
⇒ Seal the bag and refrigerate for 3 to 5 hours
⇒ Divide ingredients: onion, beef cube, green pepper, pineapple
⇒ Grill about 9 minutes each side

Nutrition Facts per Serving:
Calories: 495 kcals, **Carbohydrate:** 19g, **Protein:** 52g, **Fat:** 25g, **Sodium:** 128mg, **Potassium:** 944mg **Phosphorous:** 413mg,

Fajitas from Turkey

Diabetes-friendly
Preparation Time: 5 minutes
Cooking Time: 20 minutes
Servings: 4

Ingredients:
- o   1-pound boneless turkey breast
- o   1/4 teaspoon pepper
- o   1 teaspoon chili powder
- o   2 tablespoons lime juice
- o   1 tablespoon freshly cut coriander
- o   1 tablespoon olive oil
- o   1 cup chopped tomato
- o   1 tablespoon chopped red onion
- o   1/4 teaspoon minced garlic
- o   4 7-inch flour tortillas
- o   3 cup grated lettuce
- o   1/2 cup light sour cream

Directions:
⇒ Sprinkle the turkey with pepper, 1 clove of minced garlic, chili powder, lime juice, 1 tablespoon coriander and oil. Flip to wrap. Cover and marinate in the refrigerator for 3 hours or more.
⇒ To make the sauce, combine the tomato, 2 tablespoons of coriander, onion and 1/4 teaspoon of garlic in a small bowl. Let stand for 1 hour.
⇒ In a non-stick frying pan roast the turkey 10 cm from the heat on each side for 10 minutes. Cut into strips. While cooking, wrap the tortillas in aluminum foil and heat them in the oven for 8 minutes.
⇒ Serve the turkey, sauce, lettuce and sour cream in hot tortillas.

Nutrition Facts per Serving:
Calories: 385 kcals, **Carbohydrate:** 26g, **Protein:** 30g, **Fat:** 18g, **Sodium:** 430 mg, **Potassium:** 581mg, **Phosphorous:** 325mg.

Country Fried Steak

Preparation Time: 10 minutes
Cooking Time: 1 hour and 40 minutes
Servings: 3

Ingredients:
- o   1 tablespoon dried onion
- o   ½ cup flour
- o   1 teaspoon paprika
- o   3 tablespoons olive oil
- o   ¼ teaspoon pepper
- o   4 round steaks (2-ounce each)
- o   2 egg whites

Directions:
⇒ Trim excess fat from steak and cut into small pieces.
⇒ Combine flour, paprika and pepper and mix together. Season meat with the flour mixture.
⇒ Dip in beaten egg, then dredge in flour again.
⇒ Preheat non-stick fry pan with oil.
⇒ Cook steak on both sides (4 minutes each side)
⇒ When the color of steak is brown remove and drain on paper towels.
⇒ Serve hot and enjoy.

Nutrition Facts per Serving:
Calories: 201 kcals, **Carbohydrate:** 13g, **Protein:** 10g, **Fat:** 12g, **Sodium:** 41mg, **Potassium:** 169mg, **Phosphorous:** 88mg.

Apple Spice Pork Chops

Diabetes-friendly recipe
Preparation Time: 20 minutes
Cooking Time: 1 hour
Servings: 3

Ingredients:
- 10 oz pork chops
- 2 tablespoons butter
- 1/4 cup brown sugar
- 1/4 teaspoon salt
- 1/4 teaspoon pepper
- 1/4 teaspoon nutmeg
- 1/4 teaspoon cinnamon
- 2 medium tart apples, peeled and sliced

Directions:
⇒ Preheat the oven to 475°F
⇒ Melt butter in a non-stick frying pan and stir in brown sugar, pepper, nutmeg, cinnamon and apples. Sauté for 7 minutes, then set the sauce apart.
⇒ Trim off excess fat from the meat.
⇒ Put the pork chops in roasting pan and toss to coat with the apple sauce.
⇒ Bake for 30 minutes.
⇒ Serve and enjoy.

Nutrition Facts per Serving:
Calories: 255 kcals, **Carbohydrate:** 12g, **Protein:** 21g, **Fat:** 15g, **Sodium:** 43mg, **Potassium:** 352mg **Phosphorous:** 160mg,

Crispy Sesame Chicken

Preparation Time *2hr 20 minutes*
Cooking Time: 35 minutes
Servings: 4

Ingredients:
- 4 tablespoons sunflower oil
- 2 egg whites, lightly beaten
- 3 tablespoons cornstarch
- ¼ teaspoon ground pepper
- 2 garlic cloves, minced
- 2 teaspoons paprika
- 1 chicken breast- chopped into bite-size chunks
- 1 tablespoon rice vinegar
- 2 tablespoons honey
- 3 tablespoons tomato sauce, no salt added
- 2 tablespoons of sesame seeds
- 1 cup white rice, cooked (unsalted)

Directions:
⇒ Take a shallow small bowl, add cornstarch, pepper, paprika, 1 tablespoon of garlic and mix well.
⇒ Heat the oil in a large non-stick frying pan until very hot.
⇒ In the meanwhile place the egg whites in another shallow bowl.
⇒ Dredge the chicken in the seasoned cornstarch, then dip in the egg and dredge it once more in the seasoned cornstarch.
⇒ Add to the frying pan and cook on a medium heat for 6 minutes, stirring during cooking, until well browned.
⇒ Remove from the pan and place in a bowl lined with paper towels.
⇒ Add honey, rice vinegar, tomato sauce to the hot wok, stir and bubble over high heat until the sauce reduces by about a third (should take 2-3 minutes). Add the chicken back in and toss in the sauce to coat. Cook for 1-2 minutes.
⇒ Serve with boiled rice and top with sesame seeds

Nutrition:
Calories: 396 kcals, **Carbohydrate:** 25g, **Protein:** 20g, **Fat:** 24g, **Sodium:** 177mg, **Potassium:** 289mg **Phosphorous:** 181mg,

Garlic Chicken with Balsamic Vinegar

Diabetes-friendly recipe
Preparation Time: 5 minutes *50-50*
Cooking Time: 25 minutes
Servings: 4

Ingredients:
- 1 boneless, and skinless chicken breast
- 1 teaspoon fresh ground black pepper

- 1 tablespoon olive oil
- 1 peeled garlic clove
- ¾ cup white button mushrooms, sliced
- ¼ cup balsamic vinegar
- ¾ cup low-sodium chicken broth
- 1 bay leaf
- ¼ teaspoon thyme leaves
- 1 tablespoon cornstarch OR 2 TBLS FLOUR
- 1 cup white rice, cooked (unsalted)

Directions:

⇒ Wash the chicken breasts, trim excess fat and coat each side with pepper

⇒ Use a non-stick frying pan and heat the olive oil over medium-high heat. Cook 3 minutes.

⇒ Add in the garlic, spread the mushrooms over, and turn the chicken around to prevent it from sticking to the mushroom. Cook for 3 minutes.

⇒ Mix the balsamic vinegar, low-sodium chicken broth, thyme leaves, cornstarch and the bay leaf in a small bowl. Add the mixture to the pan with chicken, and stir until the sauce is thickened.

⇒ Cover and cook for about 10 minutes over medium-low heat.

⇒ Remove the bay leaf and serve with white rice.

Nutrition Facts per Serving:
Calories: 300 kcals, **Carbohydrate:** 44g, **Protein:** 16g, **Fat:** 6g, **Sodium:** 43mg, **Potassium:** 399mg, **Phosphorous:** 178mg.

Turkey Breast with Cranberry Gravy

Diabetes-friendly recipe
Preparation Time: 10 minutes
Cooking Time: 1 hours and 30 minutes
Servings: 6

Ingredients:
- ¼ cup onion
- ⅓ cup celery
- 2 cups carrots
- 1-pound boneless, skinless turkey breast
- 1 tablespoon olive oil
- 1 teaspoon herb seasoning (see recipe)
- 1 cup cranberry sauce

Directions:
⇒ Chop the onion, celery and carrots.
⇒ Place the whole turkey breast and the vegetables into a non-stick frying pan with oil.
⇒ Add water and herb seasoning. Cover and cook over low heat for 1 ½ hour.

⇒ Remove and slice the turkey breast, serving with the vegetables and cranberry sauce.

Nutrition Facts per Serving:
Calories: 302 kcals, **Carbohydrate:** 25g, **Protein:** 28g, **Fat:** 6g, **Sodium:** 282mg, **Potassium:** 528mg, **Phosphorous:** 257mg.

Grilled Pineapple Chicken

Preparation Time: 10 minutes
Cooking Time: 25 minutes
Servings: 4

Ingredients:
- 1 cup dry sherry
- 1 cup pineapple juice
- 1 tablespoon reduced-sodium soy sauce
- 1 pound skinless, bone-in chicken breast
- 4 pineapple rings

Directions:
⇒ Using a zip-lock bag, place in all the ingredients excluding the pineapple.
⇒ Refrigerate and marinate overnight
⇒ Using an indoor or barbecue grill, place on top of the marinated chicken. Cook for about 15 to 20 minutes or until done, and discard the unused marinade
⇒ At the last few minutes of cooking, place the pineapple on top of the grill for about 2 minutes on both sides to heat
⇒ Serve half a chicken breast per person, topped with the pineapple.

Nutrition Facts per Serving:
Calories: 278 kcals, **Carbohydrate:** 17g, **Protein:** 26g, **Fat:** 3g, **Sodium:** 174mg, **Potassium:** 683mg, **Phosphorous:** 262mg,

Chicken Enchiladas

Diabetes-friendly recipe
Preparation Time: 15 minutes
Cooking Time: 30 minutes
Servings: 4

Ingredients:
- 8 ounces boneless and skinless chicken breasts
- 1 packet reduced-sodium taco sauce mix
- ⅔ cup water — ADD MORE
- 1 cup red bell pepper, diced
- 4 (6-inch) corn tortillas
- 4 tablespoons sour cream

Directions:
⇒ Preheat oven to 350°F
⇒ Cut the chicken into strips and cook over medium-high heat in a non-stick frying pan for 10 minutes.
⇒ Mix the taco sauce in a small bowl with ⅔ cup of water
⇒ Add in the red bell pepper alongside ⅓ cup of the taco sauce into the frying pan. Cook until for 10 minutes.
⇒ Using a baking dish, spray with a non-stick cooking spray
⇒ To prepare the enchiladas, spoon out the chicken and pepper mixture over the tortillas and roll up, then place each of the enchiladas into the baking dish to hold the rolled shape. Pour the remainder of the taco sauce over the top
⇒ Bake the enchiladas for about 5 to 7 minutes or until the edges start to brown
⇒ Top each enchilada with one tablespoon of sour cream and serve hot.

Nutrition Facts per Serving:
Calories: 166 kcals, **Carbohydrate:** 17g, **Protein:** 15g, **Fat:** 5g, **Sodium:** 45mg, **Potassium:** 354mg, **Phosphorous:** 198mg.

Chapter 11. Fish and Seafood Mains

Shrimp Paella

Diabetes-friendly recipe
Preparation time: 5 minutes
Cooking time: 10 minutes
Servings: 2

Ingredients:
- 1 cup white rice, cooked
- 1 chopped red onion
- 1 tsp. paprika
- 1 chopped garlic clove
- 1 tbsp. olive oil
- 6 oz. frozen cooked shrimp
- 1 deseeded and sliced chili pepper
- 1 tablespoon dried oregano

Directions:
⇒ Heat the olive oil in a large pan on medium-high heat.
⇒ Add the onion and garlic and sauté for 2-3 minutes until soft.
⇒ Now add the shrimp and sauté for a further 5 minutes or until hot through.
⇒ Now add the herbs, spices, chili and rice with 1/2 cup boiling water.
⇒ Stir until everything is warm and the water has been absorbed.
⇒ Plate and serve.

Nutrition Facts per Serving:
Calories: 123kcals, **Carbohydrate:** 13g, **Protein:** 9g, **Fat:** 4g, **Sodium:** 313mg, **Potassium:** 128mg, **Phosphorous:** 21mg.

Herbed Shrimps

Diabetes-friendly recipe
Preparation Time: 5 minutes
Cooking Time: 0 minutes
Servings: 4

Ingredients:
- 1/2 lb. shrimp, cooked, peeled, and deveined
- 1/2 cup reduced-fat sour cream
- 2 scallions, coarsely chopped
- 1 teaspoon lemon zest, finely grated
- 2 teaspoons fresh lemon juice

Directions:
⇒ Place the minced shrimp with the sour cream in a bowl.
⇒ Add in scallions, lemon juice, and lemon zest.
⇒ Mix well and refrigerate for 1 hour.
⇒ Serve and enjoy.

Nutrition Facts per Serving:
Calories: 97 kcals, **Carbohydrate:** 3g, **Protein:** 10g, **Fat:** 5g, **Sodium:** 86mg, **Potassium:** 235mg, **Phosphorous:** 137mg

Salmon & Pesto Salad

Diabetes-friendly recipe
Preparation time: 5 minutes
Cooking time: 15 minutes
Servings: 2

Ingredients:
- 1 minced garlic clove
- ½ cup fresh arugula
- ¼ cup extra virgin olive oil
- ½ cup fresh basil
- 1 tsp. black pepper
- 4 oz. skinless salmon fillet
- ½ juiced lemon
- 4 sliced radishes
- ½ cup iceberg lettuce
- 1 tsp. black pepper

Directions:
⇒ Prepare the pesto by blending garlic, arugula, olive oil, basil, black pepper in a food processor. Set aside.
⇒ Add a non-stick frying pan to the stove on medium-high heat.
⇒ Add the salmon to the pan.
⇒ Cook for 7–8 minutes.
⇒ Stir and cook for another 3–4 minutes.
⇒ Remove fillets from the pan and allow to rest.
⇒ Mix the lettuce and the radishes and squeeze over the juice of ½ lemon.
⇒ Flake the salmon with a fork and mix through the salad.
⇒ Toss to coat and sprinkle with a little black pepper

to serve.

Nutrition Facts per Serving:
Calories: 187 kcals, **Carbohydrate:** 2g, **Protein:** 6g, **Fat:** 8g, **Sodium:** 20 mg, **Potassium:** 172mg, **Phosphorous:** 67mg.

Garlic Flavored Cod

Diabetes-friendly recipe
Preparation Time: 5 minutes
Cooking Time: 20 minutes
Servings: 4

Ingredients:
- 4 cod fillets, 6 ounces each
- ¾ pound baby bok choy halved
- 4 tablespoons olive oil
- 2 tablespoon garlic, minced
- 1 teaspoon pepper

Directions:
⇒ Preheat your oven to 400°F.
⇒ Cut 3 sheets of aluminum foil (large enough to fit fillet).
⇒ Place cod fillet on each sheet and add oil and garlic on top.
⇒ Add bok choy, season with pepper.
⇒ Fold packet and enclose them in pouches.
⇒ Arrange on the baking sheet and bake for 20 minutes.
⇒ Let it cool for 10 minutes and serve.

Nutrition Facts per Serving:
Calories: 262 kcals, **Carbohydrates:** 4g, **Protein:** 28g, **Fat:** 15g, **Sodium:** 197mg, **Potassium:** 8mg, **Phosphorus:** 1mg

Baked Fennel & Garlic Sea Bass

Diabetes-friendly recipe
Preparation time: 5 minutes
Cooking time: 15 minutes
Servings: 2

Ingredients:
- 1 lemon
- ½ sliced fennel bulb
- 6 oz. sea bass fillets
- 1 tsp. black pepper
- 2 garlic cloves

Directions:
⇒ Preheat the oven to 375°F.
⇒ Sprinkle black pepper over the Sea Bass.
⇒ Slice the fennel bulb and garlic cloves.
⇒ Add 1 salmon fillet and half the fennel and garlic to one sheet of baking paper or tin foil.
⇒ Repeat for the other fillet.
⇒ Fold and add to the oven for 15 minutes.
⇒ Squeeze in lemon and serve.

Nutrition Facts per Serving:
Calories: 99 kcals, **Carbohydrate:** 4 g, **Protein:** 12g, **Fat:** 4g, **Sodium:** 58mg, **Potassium:** 155 mg, **Phosphorous:** 20mg.

Lemon, Garlic & Cilantro Tuna and Rice

Gluten-free recipe
Preparation time: 5 minutes
Cooking time: 0 minutes
Servings: 2

Ingredients:
- ½ cup arugula
- 1 tbsp. extra virgin olive oil
- 1 cup white rice, cooked
- 1 teaspoon black pepper
- ¼ finely diced red onion
- 1 juiced lemon
- 3 oz. canned tuna
- 2 tablespoon fresh cilantro, chopped

Directions:
⇒ Mix the olive oil, pepper, cilantro, and red onion in a bowl.
⇒ Stir in the tuna and rice. Cover and refrigerate for 2 hours or serve immediately.
⇒ Sprinkle with arugula and serve.

Nutrition Facts per Serving:
Calories: 126 kcals, **Carbohydrate:** 15g, **Protein:** 6g, **Fat:** 4g, **Sodium:** 12mg, **Potassium:** 108mg, **Phosphorous:** 69mg.

Cod & Green Bean Risotto

Preparation time: 4 minutes
Cooking time: 40 minutes
Servings: 4

Ingredients:
- ½ cup arugula
- 1 white onion, finely diced
- 6 oz. cod fillet
- 1 cup white rice
- 2 lemon wedges
- 1 cup boiling water
- ¼ teaspoon black pepper

- o   1 cup low sodium chicken broth
- o   1 tablespoon extra-virgin olive oil
- o   ½ cup green beans

Directions:
⇒ In a large non-stick frying pan heat the oil over medium heat.
⇒ Sauté the chopped onion for 5 minutes until soft. Add rice and stir for 1–2 minutes.
⇒ Combine the broth with boiling water.
⇒ Add half of the liquid to the pan and stir slowly.
⇒ Slowly add the rest of the liquid whilst continuously stirring for up to 20 minutes.
⇒ Stir in the green beans to the risotto.
⇒ Place the fish on top of the rice, cover, and simmer for 5 minutes.
⇒ Sprinkle with freshly ground pepper to serve and a squeeze of fresh lemon.
⇒ Garnish with the lemon wedges and serve with the arugula.

Nutrition Facts per Serving:
Calories: 250 kcals, **Carbohydrate:** 42g, **Protein:** 10g, **Fat:** 5g, **Sodium:** 47mg, **Potassium:** 192mg, **Phosphorous:** 87mg.

Sardine Fish Cakes

Diabetes-friendly recipe
Preparation Time: 10 minutes
Cooking Time: 10 minutes
Servings: 4

Ingredients:
- o   11 oz. sardines, canned, drained
- o   1/3 cup shallot, chopped
- o   1 teaspoon chili flakes
- o   2 tablespoon wheat flour, whole grain
- o   1 egg, beaten
- o   1 teaspoon chives, chopped
- o   1 teaspoon olive oil
- o   1 teaspoon butter

Directions:
⇒ Put the butter in a non-stick frying pan and melt it.
⇒ Add shallot and cook it until translucent.
⇒ Transfer the shallot to the mixing bowl and add sardines, chili flakes, flour, egg, chives. Mix up until smooth with the help of the fork.
⇒ Make 8 medium size cakes and place them in the frying pan
⇒ Add olive oil.
⇒ Roast the fish cakes for 3 minutes from each side over medium heat.

⇒ Dry the cooked fish cakes with a paper towel if needed and transfer them in the serving plates.

Nutrition Facts per Serving:
Calories: 218 kcals, **Carbohydrate:** 5g, **Protein:** 21g, **Fat:** 12g, **Sodium:** 256mg, **Potassium:** 368mg, **Phosphorous:** 414mg.

Cajun Catfish

Diabetes-friendly
Preparation Time: 10 minutes
Cooking Time: 10 minutes
Servings: 4

Ingredients:
- o   16 oz. catfish steaks (4 oz. each fish steak)
- o   1 tablespoon Cajun spices
- o   1 egg white, beaten
- o   1 tablespoon sunflower oil

Directions:
⇒ Pour sunflower oil into a non-stick frying pan and preheat it.
⇒ Meanwhile, dip every catfish steak in the beaten egg and coat it in Cajun spices.
⇒ Place the fish steaks in the hot oil and roast them for 4 minutes from each side.
⇒ The cooked catfish steaks should have a light brown crust.
⇒ Serve and enjoy.

Nutrition Facts per Serving:
Calories: 176kcals, **Carbohydrate:** 1g, **Protein:** 18g, **Fat:** 10g, **Sodium:** 301mg, **Potassium:** 354mg, **Phosphorous:** 232mg.

Sage Salmon Fillet

Diabetes-friendly recipe
Preparation Time: 5 minutes
Cooking Time: 30 minutes
Servings: 4

Ingredients:
- o   12 oz. salmon fillet
- o   1 teaspoon sesame oil
- o   1 tablespoon sage

Directions:
⇒ Rub the fillet with sage.
⇒ Place the fish in a baking tray and spray it with sesame oil.
⇒ Cook the fish for 30 minutes at 365°F.

⇒ Serve and enjoy

Nutrition Facts per Serving:
Calories: 165 kcals, **Carbohydrate:** 1g, **Protein:** 17g, **Fat:** 11g, **Sodium:** 41mg, **Potassium:** 314mg, **Phosphorous:** 177mg.

Spanish Cod in Sauce

Diabetes-friendly recipe
Preparation Time: 10 minutes
Cooking Time: 5.5 hours
Servings: 2

Ingredients:
- 1 teaspoon tomato paste
- 1 teaspoon garlic, diced
- 1 white onion, sliced
- 1 jalapeño pepper, chopped
- 1/3 cup vegetable stock
- 14 oz. Spanish cod fillet
- 1 teaspoon paprika
- 4 bay leaves

Directions:
⇒ Pour vegetable stock into a large saucepan.
⇒ Add tomato paste and mix up the liquid until homogenous.
⇒ Add garlic, onion, jalapeno pepper, paprika. Bring the liquid to boil and then simmer it for 10 minutes.
⇒ Chop the cod fillet and add it to the tomato liquid.
⇒ Close the lid and simmer the fish for 10 minutes over low heat.
⇒ Serve the fish in bowls and garnish with bay leaves.

Nutrition Facts per Serving:
Calories: 83 kcals, **Carbohydrate:** 4g, **Protein:** 16g, **Fat:** 1g, **Sodium:** 129mg, **Potassium:** 82mg, **Phosphorous:** 14mg.

Fish Shakshuka

Diabetes-friendly recipe
Preparation Time: 5 minutes
Cooking Time: 15 minutes
Servings: 4

Ingredients:
- 2 eggs
- 2 egg whites
- 1 cup tomatoes, chopped
- 3 bell peppers, chopped
- 1 tablespoon butter
- 1 teaspoon tomato paste
- 1 teaspoon chili pepper
- 1 tablespoon fresh dill
- 12 oz. cod fillet, chopped
- 1 tablespoon scallions, chopped
- ½ teaspoon black pepper

Directions:
⇒ Melt butter in a large non-stick frying pan.
⇒ Add chili pepper, bell peppers, and tomatoes.
⇒ Sprinkle the vegetables with scallions, dill, salt, and chili pepper. Sauté for 5 minutes.
⇒ Add chopped cod fillet and stir gently.
⇒ Close the lid and simmer the ingredients for 5 minutes over medium heat.
⇒ Slightly beat eggs and egg whites in a small bowl. Season with black pepper.
⇒ Pour the beaten eggs over the fish and close the lid. Cook shakshuka with the closed lid for 5 minutes.
⇒ Serve and enjoy.

Nutrition Facts per Serving:
Calories: 163 kcals, **Carbohydrate:** 8g, **Protein:** 21g, **Fat:** 6g, **Sodium:** 130mg, **Potassium:** 375mg, **Phosphorous:** 83mg.

Salmon Baked in Foil with Fresh Thyme

Diabetes-friendly recipe
Preparation Time: 10 minutes
Cooking Time: 30 minutes
Servings: 4

Ingredients:
- 4 fresh thyme sprigs
- 4 garlic cloves, peeled, roughly chopped
- 16 oz. salmon fillets (4 oz. each fillet)
- ½ teaspoon ground black pepper
- 4 teaspoons butter
- ¼ teaspoon cumin seeds

Directions:
⇒ Line the baking tray with foil.
⇒ Sprinkle the fish fillets with ground black pepper, cumin seeds, and arrange them in the tray with oil.
⇒ Add thyme sprigs on top of every fillet.
⇒ Then add cream and garlic.
⇒ Bake the fish for 30 minutes at 345°F.

Nutrition Facts per Serving:
Calories: 251 kcals, **Carbohydrate:** 1g, **Protein:** 23g, **Fat:** 17g, **Sodium:** 56mg, **Potassium:** 443mg, **Phosphorous:** 243mg.

Poached Halibut in Lemon Sauce

Diabetes-friendly recipe
Preparation Time: 10 minutes
Cooking Time: 10 minutes
Servings: 4

Ingredients:
- 1-pound halibut
- 6 tablespoons olive oil
- 1 rosemary sprig
- ½ teaspoon ground black pepper
- 1 teaspoon honey
- ¼ cup of orange juice
- 1 teaspoon cornstarch

Directions:
⇒ Mel butter in a saucepan. Add rosemary sprig.
⇒ Pour lemon juice and add honey.
⇒ Sprinkle the halibut with ground black pepper and cornstarch.
⇒ Put the fish in the saucepan for 4 minute each side over medium heat.
⇒ Transfer the halibut to the plate and cut it on 4.
⇒ Place every fish serving on the serving plate and top with lemon sauce.

Nutrition Facts per Serving:
Calories: 304 kcals, **Carbohydrate:** 3g, **Protein:** 21g, **Fat:** 23g, **Sodium:** 78mg, **Potassium:** 516mg, **Phosphorous:** 270mg,

Fish Papillote

Diabetes-friendly recipe
Gluten- Free recipe
Preparation Time: 15 minutes
Cooking Time: 20 minutes
Servings: 3

Ingredients:
- 15 oz. snapper fillet
- 1 tablespoon fresh dill, chopped
- 1 white onion, peeled, sliced
- ½ teaspoon tarragon
- ½ teaspoon hot pepper
- 2 tablespoons sour cream
- 1 lemon, sliced

Directions:
⇒ Preheat the oven to 355°F.
⇒ Cut the snapper fillet into 3 pieces and sprinkle with tarragon, and hot pepper.
⇒ Place each FISH FILLET in the center of a 15-inch square of PARCHMENT PAPER
⇒ Top the fish with sour cream, sliced onion, and fresh dill.
⇒ Bring parchment paper size up over mixture. Double fold top and sides to seal, making packets.
⇒ Bake for 20 minutes at 355°F.
⇒ Garnish with lemon slices and serve hot.

Nutrition Facts per Serving:
Calories: 130 kcals, **Carbohydrate:** 3g, **Protein:** 22g, **Fat:** 3g, **Sodium:** 71mg, **Potassium:** 494mg, **Phosphorous:** 223mg.

Tuna Casserole

Diabetes-friendly recipe
Preparation Time: 15 minutes
Cooking Time: 35 minutes
Servings: 4

Ingredients:
- 4 tomatoes, chopped
- 12 oz. tuna filet, chopped
- 1 teaspoon ground coriander
- 1 teaspoon olive oil
- ½ teaspoon dried oregano
- 1 teaspoon hot chili

Directions:
⇒ Preheat the oven to 355°F.
⇒ Brush a casserole mold with olive oil.
⇒ Mix up together chopped tuna fillet with dried oregano, ground coriander, hot chili.
⇒ Place the fish in the mold and flatten well to get the layer.
⇒ Then add chopped tomatoes and cover the casserole with foil and secure the edges.
⇒ Bake for 35 minutes at 355°F.

Nutrition Facts per Serving:
Calories: 145 kcals, **Carbohydrate:** 5g, **Protein:** 23g, **Fat:** 21g, **Sodium:** 52mg, **Potassium:** 749mg, **Phosphorous:** 32mg.

Oregano Salmon with Crunchy Crust

Diabetes-friendly recipe
Preparation Time: 10 minutes
Cooking Time: 2 hours
Servings: 2

Ingredients:
- 10 oz. salmon fillet
- 2 tablespoons panko breadcrumbs
- 1 oz. Parmesan, grated

- o   1 teaspoon dried oregano
- o   1 teaspoon olive oil
- o   1 tablespoon fresh dill, chopped

Directions:
⇒ Preheat the oven to 385°F.
⇒ In a mixing bowl, combine together panko breadcrumbs, Parmesan, and dried oregano.
⇒ Sprinkle the salmon with olive oil and coat in the breadcrumb's mixture.
⇒ Line the baking tray with baking paper.
⇒ Place the salmon in the tray and bake salmon for 25 minutes.
⇒ Top with fresh dill and serve hot.

Nutrition Facts per Serving:
Calories: 178 kcals, **Carbohydrate:** 2g, **Protein:** 17g, **Fat:** 8g, **Sodium:** 121mg, **Potassium:** 275mg, **Phosphorous:** 197mg.

Ginger Shrimp with Snow Peas

Diabetes-friendly recipe
Preparation Time: 20 minutes
Cooking Time: 12 minutes
Servings: 4

Ingredients:
- o   2 tablespoons of extra-virgin olive oil
- o   1 tablespoon of minced peeled fresh ginger
- o   2 cups of snow peas
- o   1½ cups of frozen baby peas
- o   3 tablespoons of water
- o   1 pound of medium shrimp, shelled and deveined
- o   2 tablespoons balsamic vinegar
- o   ⅛ teaspoon of freshly ground black pepper

Directions:
⇒ In a large wok or non-stick frying pan, heat the olive oil over medium heat.
⇒ Add the ginger and stir-fry for 1 minute.
⇒ Add the snow peas and sauté for 3 minutes, until they are tender-crisp.
⇒ Add baby peas and water and stir. Cover the wok and steam for 10 minutes
⇒ Stir in the shrimp and stir-fry for 5 minutes.
⇒ Add pepper and balsamic vinegar; stir and serve.

Nutrition Facts per Serving:
Calories: 199 kcals, **Carbohydrates:** 11g, **Protein:** 20g, **Fat:** 8g, **Sodium:** 691mg, **Potassium:** 455mg, **Phosphorus:** 286mg.

Fish Chili with Lentils

Diabetes-friendly recipe
Preparation Time: 10 minutes
Cooking Time: 30 minutes
Servings: 4

Ingredients:
- o   1 red pepper, chopped
- o   1 yellow onion, diced
- o   1 teaspoon ground black pepper
- o   1 teaspoon butter
- o   1 jalapeño pepper, chopped
- o   ½ cup lentils
- o   3 cups vegetable stock
- o   1 tablespoon tomato paste
- o   1 teaspoon chili pepper
- o   3 tablespoons fresh cilantro, chopped
- o   8 oz. cod, chopped

Directions:
⇒ Put butter, red pepper, onion, and ground black pepper in a saucepan.
⇒ Sauté the vegetables for 5 minutes over medium heat.
⇒ Add chopped jalapeño pepper, lentils, chili pepper.
⇒ Mix up the mixture well and add vegetable stock and tomato paste.
⇒ Stir until homogenous. Add cod.
⇒ Close the lid and cook chili for 20 minutes over medium heat.

Nutrition Facts per Serving:
Calories: 173 kcals, **Carbohydrate:** 23g, **Protein:** 17g, **Fat:** 2g, **Sodium:** 566mg, **Potassium:** 608mg, **Phosphorous:** 211mg.

Chili Mussels

Vegetarian-friendly recipe
Preparation Time: 7 minutes
Cooking Time: 10 minutes
Servings: 4

Ingredients:
- o   1-pound mussels
- o   1 chili pepper, chopped
- o   1 cup vegetable stock
- o   1 teaspoon olive oil
- o   1 teaspoon minced garlic
- o   1 teaspoon ground coriander
- o   4 tablespoons lemon juice

Directions:
⇒ Heat oil in a large saucepan/wok over medium heat.
⇒ Add mussels, chili pepper, vegetable stock, minced garlic, ground coriander.
⇒ Cook 5 minutes or until the mussels will open the shells.
⇒ Remove it from the heat and serve with freshly squeezed lemon juice.

Nutrition Facts per Serving:
Calories: 121 kcals, **Carbohydrate:** 7g, **Protein:** 14g, **Fat:** 4g, **Sodium:** 505mg, **Potassium:** 434mg, **Phosphorous:** 233mg.

Fried Scallops in Heavy Cream

Vegetarian-friendly
Preparation Time: 10 minutes
Cooking Time: 7 minutes
Servings: 4

Ingredients:
- ½ cup light cream
- 1 teaspoon fresh rosemary
- ½ teaspoon dried cumin
- ½ teaspoon garlic, diced
- 8 oz. bay scallops
- 1 teaspoon olive oil
- ¼ teaspoon chili flakes

Directions:
⇒ Heat olive oil in a large saucepan over medium heat.
⇒ Sprinkle scallops with chili flakes, and dried cumin and place in the hot oil.
⇒ Add fresh rosemary and diced garlic.
⇒ Roast the scallops for 2 minutes from each side.
⇒ Add heavy cream and cook covered for 3 minutes.
⇒ Serve hot and enjoy.

Nutrition Facts per Serving:
Calories: 109 kcals, **Carbohydrate:** 3g, **Protein:** 8g, **Fat:** 7g, **Sodium:** 245mg, **Potassium:** 167mg, **Phosphorous:** 219mg,

Lettuce Seafood Wraps

Vegetarian-friendly recipe
Preparation Time: 10 minutes
Cooking Time: 0 minutes
Servings: 6

Ingredients:
- 4 lettuce leaves
- 8 oz. salmon, canned
- 1 cucumber
- 2 tablespoons light yogurt
- ½ teaspoon minced garlic
- 1 tablespoon fresh dill, chopped
- ¼ teaspoon tarragon

Directions:
⇒ Mash the salmon and crab meat with the help of a fork.
⇒ Add yogurt, minced garlic, fresh dill, and tarragon.
⇒ Grate the cucumber and add it to the seafood mixture. Mix up well.
⇒ Fill the lettuce leaves with the mixture.
⇒ Refrigerate for 20 minutes and serve.

Nutrition Facts per Serving:
Calories: 140 kcals, **Carbohydrate:** 13g, **Protein:** 24g, **Fat:** 3g, **Sodium:** 338mg, **Potassium:** 986mg, **Phosphorous:** 318mg.

Mango Tilapia Fillets

Diabetes-friendly recipe
Preparation Time: 10 minutes
Cooking Time: 15 minutes
Servings: 4

Ingredients:
- ¼ cup coconut flakes
- 5 oz. mango, peeled
- 13 tablespoons shallot, chopped
- 1 teaspoon ground turmeric
- 1 cup of water
- 1 bay leaf
- 12 oz. tilapia fillets
- 1 chili pepper, chopped
- 1 tablespoon olive oil
- 1 teaspoon paprika

Directions:
⇒ Blend together coconut flakes, mango, shallot, ground turmeric, and water.
⇒ Heat oil in a non-stick saucepan or wok.
⇒ Sprinkle the tilapia fillets with paprika.
⇒ Put fillets in the hot olive oil and sauté for 1 minute each side.
⇒ Add chili pepper, bay leaf, and blended mango mixture.
⇒ Close the lid and cook for 10 minutes over the medium heat.

Nutrition Facts per Serving:
Calories: 173 kcals, **Carbohydrate:** 11g, **Protein:** 18g, **Fat:** 7g, **Sodium:** 63mg, **Potassium:** 431mg, **Phosphorous:** 169mg.

Roasted Cod with Plums

Diabetes-friendly recipe
Preparation Time: 10 minutes
Cooking Time: 20 minutes
Servings: 4

Ingredients:
- 6 red plums, halved and pitted
- 1 pound cod fillets
- 3 tablespoons extra-virgin olive oil
- 2 tablespoons lemon juice, freshly squeezed
- ½ teaspoon dried thyme leaves
- ⅛ teaspoon freshly ground black pepper
- ½ cup light yogurt, for serving

Directions:
⇒ Preheat the oven to 375°F. Line a baking tray with baking paper.
⇒ Arrange the plums, cut side-up, along with the fish on the prepared baking sheet.
⇒ Add olive oil and lemon juice. Sprinkle with thyme and pepper.
⇒ Roast for 20 minutes or until the fish flakes when tested with a fork and the plums are tender.
⇒ Serve warm with yogurt on top.

Nutrition Facts per Serving:
Calories: 231 kcals, **Carbohydrates**: 12g, **Protein**: 21g, **Fat:** 12g, **Sodium:** 91mg, **Potassium:** 166mg, **Phosphorus:** 17mg.

Family Hit Curry

Diabetes-friendly recipe
Preparation Time: 10 minutes
Cooking Time: 21 minutes
Servings: 4

Ingredients:
- 1 tablespoon olive oil
- 1 onion, finely chopped
- 1 teaspoon fresh ginger, minced
- 3 garlic cloves, minced
- 1 tablespoon curry paste
- 2 cups fat-free plain Greek yogurt
- ¼ cup of water
- 1 teaspoon of sugar
- 1 pound cod fillets, cubed
- ½ pound prawns, peeled and deveined
- Freshly ground black pepper, to taste
- 2 tablespoons lemon juice, freshly squeezed
- ¼ cup fresh cilantro leaves, chopped

Directions:
⇒ In a large non-stick frying pan or wok, heat oil over medium heat.
⇒ Add onion and sauté for 5 minutes.
⇒ Add ginger, garlic, and curry paste and sauté for 1 minute.
⇒ Stir in yogurt, water, and sugar and bring to a boil over high heat.
⇒ Reduce the heat to medium-low. Simmer for about 5 minutes.
⇒ Stir in seafood and cook for about 10 minutes or till desired thickness.
⇒ Remove from heat and sprinkle with black pepper, lemon juice, and cilantro
⇒ Serve hot.

Nutrition Facts per Serving:
Calories: *249* kcals, **Carbohydrates:** *9g*, **Protein:** *39g*, **Fat:** *6g*, **Sodium:** *534mg*, **Potassium:** *358mg*, **Phosphorus:** *269mg*

Homemade Tuna Nicoise

Diabetes-friendly recipe
Preparation Time: 5 minutes
Cooking Time: 10 minutes
Servings: 4

Ingredients:
- 1 egg
- ½ cup of green beans
- 1 cucumber, sliced
- 1 lemon juice, freshly squeezed
- 1 teaspoon black pepper
- ¼ red onion, sliced
- 1 tablespoon olive oil
- 1 tablespoon capers
- 4 oz. canned tuna, drained
- 6 iceberg lettuce leaves
- 1 teaspoon fresh cilantro, chopped

Directions:
⇒ Prepare the salad by washing and slicing the lettuce, cucumber, and onion.
⇒ Add to a salad bowl.
⇒ Mix 1 tablespoon of oil with the lemon juice, cilantro, and capers for a salad dressing. Set aside.
⇒ Boil a pan of water on high heat, then lower to simmer and add the egg for 8 minutes. (Steam the green beans over the same pan in a steamer/colander for the 6 minutes.)
⇒ Remove the egg and rinse under cold water.
⇒ Peel and crumble.
⇒ Mix the tuna, salad, and dressing in a salad bowl.
⇒ Top with the crumbled hard-boil egg and serve with a sprinkle of black pepper.

Nutrition Facts per Serving:
Calories: 105 kcals,, **Carbohydrates** 5g, **Protein:** 9g **Fat:** 6g, **Sodium:** 84mg, **Potassium:** 241mg, **Phosphorus:** 108mg

Cajun Crab

Diabetes-friendly recipe
Preparation Time: 10 minutes
Cooking Time: 10 minutes
Servings: 2

Ingredients:
- 1 lemon, fresh and quartered
- 3 tablespoons of Cajun seasoning
- 2 bay leaves
- 4 snow crab legs, precooked and defrosted
- 1 teaspoon garlic powder
- 1 teaspoon ground paprika
- 1 teaspoon onion powder
- 1 teaspoon cayenne powder
- 2 tablespoons golden ghee

Directions:
⇒ Fill a large pot with salted water about halfway and bring to boil.
⇒ Squeeze half a lemon in the pot and lay remaining lemon quarters.
⇒ Add bay leaves and Cajun seasoning (garlic, paprika, onion, cayenne pepper)
⇒ Then season for 1 minute.
⇒ Add crab legs and boil for 8 minutes (make sure to keep them submerged the whole time).
⇒ Melt ghee in the microwave and use as a dipping sauce, enjoy!

Nutrition Facts per Serving:
Calories: 178 kcals, **Carbohydrates:** 3g, **Protein:** 24g, **Fat:** *7g*, **Sodium:** 872mg, **Potassium:** 58mg, **Phosphorus:** 11mg

Creamy Crab Soup

Diabetes-friendly recipe
Preparation Time: 10 minutes
Cooking Time: 20 minutes
Servings: 4

Ingredients:
- 1 tablespoon butter unsalted
- 1 cup of white onion, chopped
- ½ pound of fresh crab meat
- 2 cups of low-salt vegetable broth
- 1 cup water
- 1 cup of light cream
- 2 tablespoon cornstarch
- ⅛ tbsp. fresh dill
- 1 teaspoon black pepper

Directions:
⇒ Melt the butter in a large non-stick frying pan over medium heat.
⇒ Add the onion to the pot and sauté for 3 minutes.
⇒ Add the crab meat and sauté for 5 minutes.
⇒ Add the broth, stir and bring to a boil.
⇒ Add cornstarch and whisk to combine well. Add to the soup and increase the heat to medium-high.
⇒ Add dill and pepper and stir frequently until soup comes to a boil.
⇒ Serve hot.

Nutrition Facts per Serving:
Calories: 244kcals, **Carbohydrates:** 10g, **Protein:** 13g, **Fat:** *15g* **Sodium:** 876mg, **Potassium:** 288mg, **Phosphorus:** 197mg

Spicy Lime Shrimp

Diabetes-friendly recipe
Preparation Time: 10 minutes
Cooking Time: 5 minutes
Servings: 4

Ingredients:
- 1 pound shrimps, peeled and deveined
- ¼ cup of lime juice
- 1 garlic clove, minced
- 1 green onion, sliced
- 3 tbsp. of red bell pepper, diced
- 2 tbsp. of fresh cilantro, chopped
- 1 tbsp. of jalapeno chili, minced
- 1 big cucumber, sliced

Directions:
⇒ In a mixing bowl make a marinade combining lime juice, green onion, jalapeno chili, cilantro, garlic, and oil.
⇒ In a separate mixing bowl, add the shrimps with 3 tablespoons of the lime juice marinade. Cover and refrigerate for 40 minutes.
⇒ Turn on your oven's broiler. Discard the shrimp from the lime marinade and broil for around 3–4 minutes in total or 2 minutes on each side.
⇒ Plate the shrimps and pour the remaining marinade on top.
⇒ Place over the cucumber slices and serve cold.

Nutrition Facts per Serving:
Calories: 92 kcals, **Carbohydrates:** 4g, **Protein:** 16g, **Fat:** 1g, **Sodium:** 637mg, **Potassium:** 425mg, **Phosphorus:** 262mg

Seafood Casserole

Preparation Time: 20 minutes
Cooking Time: 45 minutes
Servings: 4

Ingredients:
- 2 cups eggplant, peeled and diced into 1-inch pieces
- Butter, for greasing the baking sheet
- 1 tablespoon olive oil

- ½ sweet onion, chopped
- 1 tablespoon garlic, minced
- 1 stalk celery, chopped
- ½ red bell pepper, boiled and chopped
- 3 tablespoons freshly squeezed lemon juice
- 1 tablespoon hot sauce
- ½ cup white rice, cooked
- 1 large egg
- 4 ounces shrimps, cooked
- 6 ounces crab meat, cooked

Directions:
⇒ Preheat the oven to 350°F.
⇒ Grease a 9-by-13-inch baking sheet with butter and set aside.
⇒ Heat the olive oil in a large saucepan over medium heat.
⇒ Sauté the garlic, onion, celery, eggplant and bell pepper for 5 minutes.
⇒ Add the sautéed vegetables to the eggplant, along with the lemon juice, hot sauce, seasoning, rice, and egg.
⇒ Stir to combine.
⇒ Add in shrimps, crab meat and rice.
⇒ Spoon the mixture into a casserole dish, patting down the top.
⇒ Bake for 30 minutes or until casserole is heated through and rice is tender.
⇒ Serve warm.

Nutrition Facts per Serving:
Calories: 238 kcals, **Carbohydrates:** 25g, **Protein:** 15g, **Fat:** 9g, **Sodium:** 519mg, **Potassium:** 387mg, **Phosphorus:** 231mg.

Tilapia Ceviche

Preparation Time: 15 minutes
Cooking Time: 5 minutes
Servings: 4

Ingredients:
- 1 pound of fresh tilapia fillets
- 1 cup of red onion, chopped
- ½ cup of red bell pepper, chopped
- ¼ cup of cilantro, chopped
- 1 cup of pineapple, diced
- 2 tablespoons of olive oil
- ¼ teaspoon of black pepper
- 1¼ cups of fresh lime juice
- 16 unsalted crackers

Directions:
⇒ Cube the tilapia into small chunks.
⇒ In a wok, broil tilapia cubes over high heat for about 3 minutes on each side.
⇒ Cool the tilapia for about 5 minutes, then pour the fresh lime juice on top of it, mixing properly. Ensure all tilapia pieces are coated completely with the lime juice.
⇒ Combine and mix bell pepper, onion, pineapple, cilantro, black pepper, and the olive oil with the broiled tilapia mixture.
⇒ Cover and refrigerate to marinate for about 2 hours.
⇒ Use 4 crackers with the unsalted tops for each serving.

Nutrition Facts per Serving:
Calories: 363 kcals, **Carbohydrates:** 35g, **Protein:** 26g, **Fat:** 14g, **Sodium:** 268 mg, **Potassium:** 693mg, **Phosphorus:** 316mg

Fish Tacos

Preparation Time: 10 minutes
Cooking Time: 35 minutes
Servings: 4

Ingredients:
- 1½ cup cabbage, shredded
- ½ cup of red onion, chopped
- ½ bunch cilantro, chopped
- 1 garlic clove, minced
- 2 limes
- 1 pound cod fillets
- ½ teaspoon ground cumin
- ½ teaspoon chili powder
- ¼ teaspoon black pepper
- 1 tablespoon olive oil
- ¼ cup sour cream
- 2 tablespoons skimmed milk
- 12 (6-inch) corn tortillas

Directions:
⇒ Place fish fillets on a dish and squeeze half a lime juice over it.
⇒ Sprinkle the fish fillets with the minced garlic, cumin, black pepper, chili powder, and olive oil. Toss to coat with the marinade, then refrigerate for 30 minutes.
⇒ Prepare salsa Blanca by mixing the milk, sour cream, and the other half of the lime juice. Stir to combine, and then place in the refrigerator to chill.
⇒ Broil in oven, and cover the broiler pan with aluminum foil. Broil the coated fish fillets for 10 minutes.
⇒ Heat the corn tortillas in a pan, one at a time until they become soft and warm, then wrap in a dish towel to keep them warm.
⇒ To assemble the tacos, place a piece of the fish on the tortilla, topping with the salsa Blanca, cabbage, cilantro, red onion, and the lime wedges.
⇒ Serve and enjoy.

Nutrition Facts per Serving:
Calories: 369 kcals, **Carbohydrates:** 47g, **Protein:** 27g, *Fat:* 9g, **Sodium:** 141mg, **Potassium:** 193mg, **Phosphorus:** 44mg

Chapter 12. Vegetarian Mains

Grilled Squash

Vegetarian-friendly recipe
Preparation Time: 10 minutes
Cooking Time: 6 minutes
Servings: 4

Ingredients:
- 4 zucchinis, rinsed, drained and sliced
- 4 crookneck squash, rinsed, drained and sliced
- Cooking spray
- 1/4 teaspoon garlic powder
- 1/4 teaspoon black pepper

Directions
⇒ Arrange squash on a baking sheet.
⇒ Spray with oil.
⇒ Season with garlic powder and pepper.
⇒ Grill for 3 minutes per side or until tender but not too soft.

Nutrition Facts per Serving:
Calories: 84 kcals, **Carbohydrates:** 13g, **Protein:** 5g, **Fat:** 3g, **Sodium:** 33mg, **Potassium:** 1027mg, **Phosphorus:** 150mg

Delicious Vegetarian Lasagna

Vegetarian-friendly recipe
Preparation time: 10 minutes
Cooking time: 1 hour
Servings: 4

Ingredients:
- 1 teaspoon basil
- 1 tablespoon olive oil
- ½ red pepper, sliced
- 6 lasagna sheets
- ½ red onion, diced
- ¼ teaspoon black pepper
- 1 cup rice milk
- 1 garlic clove, minced
- 1 cup eggplant, sliced
- ½ zucchini, sliced
- 1 teaspoon oregano

Directions:
⇒ Preheat oven to 325°F/Gas Mark 3.
⇒ Slice zucchini, eggplant and pepper into vertical strips.
⇒ Add the rice milk and tofu to a food processor and blitz until smooth. Set aside.
⇒ Heat the oil in a non-stick frying pan over medium heat. Add onion and garlic and sauté for 5 minutes.
⇒ Sprinkle in the herbs, pepper, eggplant, zucchini and stir through for 10 minutes.
⇒ Into a lasagna or suitable oven dish, layer 2 lasagna sheets, then 1/3 of vegetables.
⇒ Repeat for the next 2 layers, finishing with the white sauce.
⇒ Add to the oven for 50 minutes.
⇒ Serve hot and enjoy.

Nutrition Facts per Serving:
Calories: 187 kcals, **Carbohydrates:** 32g, **Protein:** 5g, **Fat:** 5g, **Sodium:** 27mg, **Potassium:** 196mg, **Phosphorus:** 58mg

Chili Tofu Noodles

Vegetarian-friendly recipe
Preparation time: 5 minutes
Cooking Time: 15 minutes
Servings: 4

Ingredients:
- ½ chili, diced red
- 2 cups rice noodles
- ½ juiced lime
- 6 ounce silken firm tofu, pressed and cubed
- 1 teaspoon fresh ginger, grated
- 1 tablespoon coconut oil
- 1 cup green beans
- 1 minced garlic clove

Directions:
⇒ Steam the green beans for 10 minutes.
⇒ Cook the noodles in a pot of boiling water for according to package directions.
⇒ Meanwhile, heat a wok over high heat and add coconut oil.
⇒ Now add tofu, chili flakes, garlic and ginger and sauté for 5 minutes.
⇒ Drain in the noodles along with the green beans and lime juice.
⇒ Toss to coat and serve hot.

Nutrition Facts per Serving:

Calories: 247 kcals, **Carbohydrates:** 44g, **Protein:** 6g, **Fat:** 5g, **Sodium:** 95mg, **Potassium:** 172mg, **Phosphorus:** 116mg

Curried Cauliflower

Vegetarian-friendly recipe
Preparation time: 5 minutes
Cooking time: 20 minutes
Servings: 4

Ingredients:
- 1 teaspoon turmeric
- 1 onion, diced
- 1 tablespoon fresh cilantro, minced
- 1 teaspoon cumin
- ½ chili, minced
- ½ cup water
- 1 garlic clove, minced
- 1 tablespoon coconut oil
- 1 teaspoon curry
- 2 cups cauliflower florets

Directions
⇒ Add the oil to a non-stick frying pan over medium heat.
⇒ Sauté the onion and garlic for 5 minutes until soft.
⇒ Add in cumin and turmeric and stir to release the aromas.
⇒ Add chili to the pan along with the cauliflower.
⇒ Stir to coat.
⇒ Pour in the water and reduce the heat to a simmer for 15 minutes.
⇒ Garnish with cilantro to serve.

Nutrition Facts per Serving:
Calories: 66 kcals, **Carbohydrates:** 7g, **Protein:** 2g, **Fat:** 19g, **Sodium:** 4mg, **Potassium:** 20mg, **Phosphorus:** 222mg

Elegant Veggie Tortillas

Vegetarian-friendly recipe
Preparation Time: 30 minutes
Cooking Time: 15 minutes
Servings: 6

Ingredients:
- 1½ cups, broccoli florets, chopped
- 1½ cups cauliflower florets, chopped
- 1 tablespoon water
- 2 teaspoons corn oil
- 1½ cups onion, chopped
- 1 garlic clove, minced
- 1 cup egg whites
- Freshly ground black pepper, to taste
- 4 7-inches corn tortillas

Directions:
⇒ In a microwave bowl, place broccoli, cauliflower, water, and microwave, covered for about 3-5 minutes.
⇒ Remove from microwave and drain any liquid.
⇒ In a wok or a non-stick frying pan heat oil over medium heat.
⇒ Add onion and sauté for 5 minutes.
⇒ Add garlic and then sauté for 1 minute.
⇒ Stir in broccoli, cauliflower and black pepper.
⇒ Reduce the heat and simmer for 10 minutes.
⇒ Remove from heat and keep aside to cool slightly.
⇒ Place broccoli mixture over ¼ of each tortilla.
⇒ Fold the outside edges inward and roll up like a burrito.
⇒ Secure each tortilla with toothpicks to secure the filling.
⇒ Cut each tortilla in half and serve.

Nutrition Facts per Serving:
Calories: 148 kcals, **Carbohydrates:** 21g, **Protein:** 10g, **Fat:** 19g, **Sodium:** 132 mg, **Potassium:** 406mg, **Phosphorus:** 137mg

Sweet and Sour Chickpeas

Vegetarian-friendly recipe
Preparation Time: 10 minutes
Cooking Time: 12 Minutes
Servings: 6

Ingredients:
- 2 tablespoons extra-virgin olive oil
- 1 onion, chopped
- 1 (14-ounce) can tropical fruit in fruit juice, strained, without juice
- ½ cup water
- 1 tablespoon honey
- 2 tablespoons lemon juice, freshly squeezed
- 2 tablespoons cornstarch
- 1 (15-ounce) no-salt-added chickpeas, drained and rinsed

Directions:
⇒ In a large saucepan, heat the olive oil over medium heat.
⇒ Sauté the onion for 4 to 5 minutes, stirring frequently, until tender.

- ⇒ In a medium bowl, whisk together water, lemon juice, honey and cornstarch.
- ⇒ When the onion is tender, add the chickpeas and cook for 5 minutes, stirring until hot.
- ⇒ Add the juice mixture and cook, stirring frequently, until the liquid is thickened, about 2 minutes.
- ⇒ Add the drained fruits to the saucepan and simmer for 2 minutes.
- ⇒ Serve and enjoy.

Nutrition Facts per Serving:
Calories: 254 kcals, **Carbohydrates**: 39g, **Protein**: 6g, **Fat:** 9g, **Sodium:** 32mg, **Potassium:** 354mg, **Phosphorus:** 23mg

Cabbage-Stuffed Mushrooms

Vegetarian-friendly recipe
Preparation Time: 20 minutes
Cooking Time: 25 Minutes
Servings: 4

Ingredients:
- 4 Portobello mushrooms
- 2 tablespoons extra-virgin olive oil
- 1 onion, chopped
- 1 teaspoon fresh ginger, minced
- 2 cups red cabbage, shredded
- ⅛ teaspoon freshly ground black pepper
- 3 tablespoons water
- 1 cup Monterey Jack cheese, shredded

Directions:
- ⇒ Preheat the oven to 400°F.
- ⇒ Rinse the mushrooms briefly and pat dry. Remove the stems and discard. Using a spoon, scrape out the dark gills on the underside of the mushroom cap. Set aside.
- ⇒ In a medium non-stick frying pan heat the olive oil over medium heat. Sauté onion and ginger for 3 minutes, stirring, until fragrant.
- ⇒ Add cabbage and pepper and sauté for 3 minutes, stirring frequently.
- ⇒ Add water, cover, and steam the cabbage for 5 minutes.
- ⇒ Remove the vegetables from the pan and place in a medium bowl; let cool for 10 minutes, then stir in the cheese.
- ⇒ Place the caps on a baking sheet and divide the filling among the mushrooms. Bake for 15 minutes.
- ⇒ Serve and enjoy.

Nutrition Facts per Serving:
Calories: 208 kcals, **Carbohydrates**: 8g, **Protein:** 9g, **Fat:** 16g, **Sodium:** 195mg, **Potassium:** 300mg, **Phosphorus:** 63mg

Curried Veggie Stir-Fry

Vegetarian-friendly recipe
Preparation Time: 20 minutes
Cooking Time: 10 Minutes
Servings: 4

Ingredients:
- 2 tablespoons extra-virgin olive oil
- 1 onion, chopped
- 4 garlic cloves, minced
- 4 cups frozen stir-fry vegetables
- 1 cup canned unsweetened full-fat coconut milk
- 1 cup water
- 2 tablespoons green curry paste

Directions:
- ⇒ In a wok or non-stick frying pan, heat the olive oil over medium-high heat. Stir-fry the onion and garlic for 3 minutes, until fragrant.
- ⇒ Add the frozen stir-fry vegetables and continue to cook for 10 minutes longer.
- ⇒ Meanwhile, in a small bowl, combine coconut milk, water, and curry paste. Stir until the paste dissolves.
- ⇒ Add the broth mixture to the wok and cook for another 5 minutes, or until the sauce has reduced slightly and all the vegetables are crisp-tender.
- ⇒ Serve over couscous or hot cooked rice.

Nutrition Facts per Serving:
Calories: 260 kcals, **Carbohydrates**: 19g, **Protein:** 4g, **Fat:** 20g, **Sodium:** 387mg, **Potassium:** 177mg, **Phosphorus:** 67mg

Creamy Mushroom Pasta

Vegetarian-friendly recipe
Preparation Time: 10 minutes
Cooking Time: 20 Minutes
Servings: 6

Ingredients:
- 12 ounces whole-grain fettuccine pasta
- 3 tablespoons extra-virgin olive oil
- 1 (8-ounce) package button mushrooms, sliced

- 2 garlic cloves, sliced
- 1 cup light cream
- 1 teaspoon ground black pepper

Directions:
⇒ In a large heavy saucepan, heat the olive oil on medium-high heat. Add the mushrooms in a single layer. Cook for 3 minutes or until the mushrooms are golden brown on one side. Carefully turn the mushrooms and cook for another 2 minutes.
⇒ Reduce the heat to medium and add the garlic. Sauté, stirring, for 2 minutes longer, until the garlic is fragrant.
⇒ Add the cream to the pan with the mushrooms and season with salt and pepper. Simmer for 3 minutes or until the mixture starts to thicken. Set aside.
⇒ Bring a large pot of water to a boil. Add pasta and cook for 7 minutes, until al dente. Drain, reserving about ⅓ cup of the pasta water,
⇒ Add the drained pasta to the pan and coat using tongs. Add the reserved pasta water if necessary, to loosen the sauce.
⇒ Serve hot.

Nutrition Facts per Serving:
Calories: 475 kcals, **Carbohydrates:** 52g, **Protein:** 12g, **Fat:** 25g, **Sodium:** 50mg, **Potassium:** 300mg, **Phosphorus:** 59mg

Chinese Tempeh Stir Fry

Vegetarian-friendly recipe
Preparation time: 5 minutes
Cooking time: 15 minutes
Servings: 2

Ingredients:
- 2 oz. tempeh, sliced
- 1 cup white rice, cooked
- 1 garlic clove, minced
- ½ cup green onions
- 1 tsp. minced fresh ginger
- 1 tbsp. coconut oil
- ½ cup corn

Directions:
⇒ Heat the oil in a wok over high heat and add garlic and ginger.
⇒ Sauté for 1 minute.
⇒ Now add the tempeh and cook for 5-6 minutes before adding the corn for a further 10 minutes.
⇒ Add the green onions and serve over white rice.

Nutrition Facts per Serving:
Calories: 120 kcals, **Carbohydrates:** 15g, **Protein:** 5g, **Fat:** 5g, **Sodium:** 105 mg, **Potassium:** 151mg, **Phosphorus:** 63mg

Broccoli with Garlic Butter and Almonds

Vegetarian-friendly recipe
Preparation Time: 10 minutes
Cooking Time: 50 minutes
Servings: 3

Ingredients:
- 1 pound fresh broccoli, cut into bite size pieces
- ¼ cup olive oil
- ½ tablespoon honey
- 1 tablespoon soy sauce
- ¼ teaspoon ground black pepper
- 2 cloves garlic, minced
- ¼ cup chopped almonds

Directions:
⇒ Put broccoli into a large pot with about 1 inch of water in the bottom. Drain, and arrange broccoli on a serving platter.
⇒ Heat the oil in a small saucepan over medium heat. Mix in the honey, soy sauce, pepper and garlic.
⇒ Bring to a boil, then remove from the heat.
⇒ Mix in the almonds and pour the sauce over the broccoli.
⇒ Serve immediately.

Nutrition Facts per Serving:
Calories: 220 kcals, **Carbohydrates:** 12g, **Protein:** 5g, **Fat:** 18g, **Sodium:** 268mg, **Potassium:** 425mg, **Phosphorus:** 116mg

Eggplant French Fries

Vegetarian-friendly recipe
Diabetes-friendly recipe
Preparation Time: 10 minutes
Cooking Time: 50 minutes
Servings: 4

Ingredients:
- 1 medium eggplant
- 2 egg whites
- ¼ cup cornstarch
- ¼ cup dry unseasoned breadcrumbs
- ½ cup olive oil
- ½ tablespoon pepper

Directions:
⇒ Peel and slice eggplant into 3/4-inch sticks, 4-inch long. Rinse and pat dry.
⇒ In a medium bowl, mix milk and egg whites until well blended.
⇒ Heat oil in a frying pan over high heat.
⇒ Add oil, stirring regularly and fry for 5 minutes.
⇒ Drain on paper towels and serve immediately.

Nutrition Facts per Serving:
Calories: 344 kcals, **Carbohydrates**: 18g, **Protein:** 4g, **Fat:** 19g, **Sodium:** 118mg, **Potassium:** 236mg, **Phosphorus:** 26mg

Thai Tofu Broth

Vegetarian-friendly
Preparation time: 5 minutes
Cooking time: 15 minutes
Servings: 4

Ingredients:
o 1 cup rice noodles
o ½ sliced onion
o 6 oz. drained, pressed and cubed tofu
o ¼ cup sliced scallions
o ½ cup water
o ½ cup canned water chestnuts
o ½ cup rice milk
o 1 tbsp. lime juice
o 1 tbsp. coconut oil
o ½ finely sliced chili
o 1 cup snow peas

Directions:
⇒ Heat the oil in a wok over high heat and then sauté the tofu until brown on each side.
⇒ Add onion and sauté for 2-3 minutes.
⇒ Add rice milk and water to the wok and bring to a boil.
⇒ Lower to medium heat and add noodles, chili and water chestnuts.
⇒ Allow to simmer for 15 minutes and then add the sugar snap peas.
⇒ Cook over medium heat for 5 minutes.
⇒ Serve with a sprinkle of scallions.

Nutrition Facts per Serving:
Calories: 190 kcals, **Carbohydrates**: 28g, **Protein:** 6g, **Fat:** 6g, **Sodium:** 64mg, **Potassium:** 159mg, **Phosphorus:** 106mg

Broccoli Steaks

Vegetarian-friendly recipe
Preparation Time: 10 minutes
Cooking Time: 25 minutes
Servings: 2

Ingredients:
o 1 medium head broccoli
o 3 tablespoons olive oil
o ¼ teaspoon garlic powder
o ¼ teaspoon onion powder
o ¼ teaspoon pepper

Directions:
⇒ Preheat the oven to 400°F. Put parchment paper on a roasting pan.
⇒ Trim the leaves off the broccoli and cut off the bottom of the stem. Cut the broccoli head in half. Cut each half into 1 to 3/4-inch slices, leaving the core in place. Cut off the smaller ends of the broccoli and save for another recipe. There should be 4 broccoli steaks.
⇒ Mix oil, garlic powder, onion powder and pepper.
⇒ Lay the broccoli on the parchment lined baking sheet.
⇒ Using half of the oil mixture, brush onto the broccoli. Bake for 20 minutes.
⇒ Remove from the oven and flip the steaks over.
⇒ Brush the steaks with remaining oil and roast for about 20 more minutes, until they are golden brown on the edges.
⇒ Serve hot or warm.

Nutrition Facts per Serving:
Calories: 109 kcals, **Carbohydrates**: 3g, **Protein:** 1g, **Fat:** 11g, **Sodium:** 13mg, **Potassium:** 125mg, **Phosphorus:** 26mg

Roasted Garlic Lemon Cauliflower

Vegetarian-friendly recipe
Diabetes- friendly recipe
Preparation Time: 10 minutes
Cooking Time: 15 minutes
Servings: 4

Ingredients:
o 1 head cauliflower, separated into florets
o 2 teaspoons olive oil
o ½ teaspoon ground black pepper
o 1 clove garlic, minced
o ½ teaspoon lemon juice

Directions:
⇒ Preheat the oven to 400 degrees F.
⇒ Bake in the preheated oven until florets are tender enough to pierce the stems with a fork, 15 to 20 minutes.
⇒ Remove and transfer to a serving platter.

Nutrition Facts per Serving:
Calories: 59 kcals, **Carbohydrates:** 8g, **Protein:** 3g, **Fat:** 3g, **Sodium:** 47mg, **Potassium:** 444mg, **Phosphorus:** *65mg*

Veg Stew

Vegetarian-friendly
Preparation time: 5 minutes
Cooking time: 35 -40 minutes
Servings: 4

Ingredients:
o 1 garlic clove
o 1 cup white rice
o 1 teaspoon ground cumin
o 1 onion, diced
o 2 cups water
o 4 turnips, peeled and diced
o 1 teaspoon cayenne pepper
o ¼ cup chopped fresh parsley
o ½ teaspoon ground cinnamon
o 2 tablespoons olive oil
o 1 teaspoon ground ginger
o 2 carrots, peeled and diced

Directions:
⇒ In a large pot, heat the oil over medium heat and sauté onion for 5 minutes, until soft.
⇒ Add the turnips and sauté for 10 minutes.
⇒ Add garlic, cumin, ginger, cinnamon, and cayenne pepper, cooking for a further 3 minutes.
⇒ Add carrots and stock to the pot and then bring to a boil.
⇒ Switch to low heat and simmer for 20 minutes.
⇒ Meanwhile add the rice to a pot of water and bring to the boil.
⇒ Turn down to simmer for 15 minutes.
⇒ Drain and place the lid on for 5 minutes to steam.
⇒ Serve the vegetables on top of the rice and enjoy.

Nutrition Facts per Serving:
Calories: *297* kcals, **Carbohydrates:** 52g, **Protein:** 5g, **Fat:** 8g, **Sodium:** 112mg, **Potassium:** 474mg, **Phosphorus:** 113mg

Couscous with Vegetables

Vegetarian-friendly
Preparation Time: 10 minutes
Cooking Time: 15 minutes
Servings: 5

Ingredients:
o 1 tablespoon butter
o ½ cup frozen peas
o ½ cup onion, minced
o ¼ cup mushrooms, sliced
o ½ cup couscous, uncooked
o 1 garlic clove, minced
o 2 tablespoons dry white wine
o ½ teaspoon dried basil
o ¼ teaspoon black pepper

Directions:
⇒ Melt the butter in a skillet over a medium high heat.
⇒ Sauté peas, onion, mushrooms, garlic and wine.
⇒ Add the herbs.
⇒ Prepare the couscous according to package instructions.
⇒ Mix the vegetables with the hot couscous and serve.

Nutrition Facts per Serving:
Calories: 135 kcals, **Carbohydrates:** 21g, **Protein:** 4g, **Fat:** 19g, **Sodium:** 22mg, **Potassium:** 116mg, **Phosphorus:** 64mg

Grill Thyme Corn on the Cob

Vegetarian-friendly
Preparation Time: 10 minutes
Cooking Time: 20 minutes
Servings: 4

Ingredients:
o 1 tablespoon grated Parmesan cheese
o 4 half-ear size frozen corn on the cob
o ½ teaspoon dried thyme
o ¼ teaspoon black pepper
o 2 tablespoon olive oil

Directions:
⇒ In a small bowl, mix the oil, cheese, thyme and black pepper.
⇒ Coat the corn in the oil mixture.
⇒ Place the corn in a foil packet topped with 2 ice cubes.

⇒ Place the corn on a grill and cook for approximately 20 minutes.
⇒ Serve and enjoy.

Nutrition Facts per Serving:
Calories: 159 kcals, **Carbohydrates:** 19g, **Protein:** 3g, **Fat:** 8g, **Sodium:** 15mg, **Potassium:** 5mg, **Phosphorus:** 9mg

Ginger Glazed Carrots

Vegetarian-friendly
Preparation Time: 10 minutes
Cooking Time: 20 minutes
Servings: 4

Ingredients:
- 2 cups carrots, sliced into 1-inch pieces
- ¼ cup apple juice
- 2 tablespoons butter
- ¼ cup boiling water
- 1 tablespoon sugar
- 1 teaspoon cornstarch
- ¼ teaspoon ground ginger

Directions:
⇒ Boil carrots until tender.
⇒ Mix sugar, cornstarch, salt, ginger, apple juice and butter.
⇒ Pour mixture over carrots and cook for 10 minutes until thickened.
⇒ Serve and enjoy.

Nutrition Facts per Serving:
Calories: 96 kcals, **Carbohydrates:** 11g, **Protein:** 1g, **Fat:** 6g, **Sodium:** 44mg, **Potassium:** 215mg, **Phosphorus:** 24mg

Sautéed Green Beans

Vegetarian-friendly
Preparation Time: 10 minutes
Cooking Time: 15 minutes
Servings: 4

Ingredients:
- 2 cup frozen green beans
- ½ cup red bell pepper
- 4 teaspoons butter
- ¼ cup onion
- 1 teaspoon dried dill weed
- ¼ tsp. black pepper

Directions:
⇒ Cook green beans in a large pan of boiling water until tender, then drain.
⇒ While the beans are cooking, melt the butter in a non-stick frying pan and sauté the other vegetables.
⇒ Add beans to sautéed vegetables.
⇒ Sprinkle with freshly ground pepper.
⇒ Serve and enjoy.

Nutrition Facts per Serving:
Calories: *66 kcals,* **Carbohydrates:** *7g,* **Protein:** *2g,* **Fat:** *4g,* **Sodium:** *4mg,* **Potassium:** *176mg,* **Phosphorus:** *30mg*

Carrot-Apple Casserole

Vegetarian-friendly
Preparation Time: 20 minutes
Cooking Time: 50 minutes
Servings: 4

Ingredients:
- 6 large carrots, peeled and sliced
- 4 large apples, peeled and sliced
- 2 tbsp. butter
- ½ cup apple juice
- 2 tbsp. all-purpose flour
- 2 tbsp. brown sugar
- ½ tsp. ground nutmeg

Directions:
⇒ Preheat oven to 350°F.
⇒ Boil carrots and apples for 5 minutes or until tender. Drain and arrange them in a large casserole dish.
⇒ Mix the flour, brown sugar and nutmeg together in a small bowl.
⇒ Rub in butter to make a crumb topping.
⇒ Sprinkle the crumb over the carrots and apples then drizzle with juice.
⇒ Bake for 50 minutes or until bubbling and golden brown.
⇒ Serve hot and enjoy.

Nutrition Facts per Serving:
Calories: 223 kcals, **Carbohydrates:** 44g, **Protein:** 2g, **Fat:** 6g, **Sodium:** 67mg, **Potassium:** 502mg, **Phosphorus:** 61mg

Broccoli-Onion Latkes

Vegetarian-friendly
Preparation Time: 20 minutes
Cooking Time: 15 minutes
Servings: 4

Ingredients:
- 3 cups broccoli florets, diced
- ½ cup onion, chopped

- o 2 large eggs, beaten
- o 2 tbsp. all-purpose white flour
- o 2 tbsp. olive oil

Directions:
⇒ Steam broccoli for 10 minutes or until tender. Drain.
⇒ Mix the flour into the eggs.
⇒ Combine the onion, broccoli and egg mixture and stir through.
⇒ Heat olive oil in a large non-stick frying pan over medium heat.
⇒ Drop a ladle of the mixture onto the pan to make 4 latkes.
⇒ Fry for a few minutes on each side until golden brown.
⇒ Drain on a paper towel and serve.

Nutrition Facts per Serving:
Calories: 133 kcals, **Carbohydrates:** 8g, **Protein:** 5g, **Fat:** 9g, **Sodium:** 50mg, **Potassium:** 299mg, **Phosphorus:** 88mg

Eggplant Casserole

Vegetarian-friendly
Preparation Time: 15 minutes
Cooking Time: 20 minutes
Servings: 3

Ingredients:
- o 3 cups eggplant
- o 2 large eggs
- o ½ teaspoon pepper
- o ¼ teaspoon sage
- o ½ cup white breadcrumbs
- o 1 tablespoon olive oil

Directions:
⇒ Preheat oven to 350°F.
⇒ Peel and cut up eggplant. Place eggplant pieces in a pan, cover with water and boil until tender. Drain and mash.
⇒ Combine beaten eggs, salt, pepper and sage with mashed eggplant. Place in a greased casserole dish.
⇒ Mix olive oil with white breadcrumbs.
⇒ Top casserole with breadcrumbs and bake 20 minutes or until top begin to brown.
⇒ Serve and enjoy.

Nutrition Facts per Serving:
Calories: 174 kcals, **Carbohydrates:** 21g, **Protein:** 7g, **Fat:** 7g, **Sodium:** 208mg, **Potassium:** 222mg, **Phosphorus:** 98mg

Asparagus Quiche

Vegetarian-friendly
Preparation Time: 15 minutes
Cooking Time: 45 minutes
Servings: 4

Ingredients:
- o 2 eggs
- o 2 egg whites
- o 1 cup cottage cheese
- o ½ tablespoon dried thyme
- o ¼ cup water
- o 8 oz. asparagus, cut into 1-inch pieces
- o ¼ teaspoon black pepper

Directions:
⇒ Preheat the oven to 375°F.
⇒ Spray baking dish with cooking spray and set aside.
⇒ Add water into the large cooking pot and bring to a boil.
⇒ Add asparagus into the boiling water and cook for 5 minutes.
⇒ Drain and rinse with cold water. In a large mixing bowl, whisk together egg whites, eggs, cottage cheese, thyme, water, pepper.
⇒ Pour egg mixture into the prepared baking dish. Sprinkle asparagus pieces into the egg mixture.
⇒ Bake for 30 minutes.
⇒ Slice & serve.

Nutrition Facts per Serving:
Calories: 91 kcals, **Carbohydrates:** 5g, **Protein:** 11g, **Fat:** 4g, **Sodium:** 247mg, **Potassium:** 216mg, **Phosphorus:** 144mg

Spinach Egg Bake

Vegetarian-friendly
Preparation Time: 15 minutes
Cooking Time: 25 minutes
Servings: 4
Ingredients:
- o 3 eggs, beaten
- o 1 teaspoon spike seasoning
- o 1/3 cup green onion, sliced
- o 1 cup mozzarella
- o 1 teaspoon olive oil
- o 3 oz fresh spinach, cooked
- o Pepper, to taste

Directions:
⇒ Preheat the oven to 375 F.
⇒ Grease casserole dish and set aside.
⇒ Heat oil in a large non-stick frying pan over medium heat.

⇒ In a large bowl mix beaten eggs, spike seasoning, pepper and spinach
⇒ Transfer the mixture into the casserole dish and spread well.
⇒ Add mozzarella and bake for 20 minutes.
⇒ Slice & serve.

Nutrition Facts per Serving :
Calories: 150 kcals, **Carbohydrates**: 2g, **Protein:** 12g, **Fat:** 11g, **Sodium:** 261mg, **Potassium:** 262mg, **Phosphorus:** 178mg

Vegetarian Quinoa Chili

Vegetarian-friendly
Preparation Time: 15 minutes
Cooking Time: 1 hour and 40 minutes
Servings: 4
Ingredients:
- ½ cup quinoa
- 3 cups vegetable broth
- ½ teaspoon chili flakes
- 1 teaspoon ground coriander.
- 1 tablespoon paprika
- 1 tablespoon cumin
- 1 tablespoon chili powder
- 8 oz chili beans, canned
- 4 oz tomato sauce
- 3 oz fire-roasted tomatoes
- 2 garlic cloves, minced
- 1 red bell pepper, chopped
- 1 poblano pepper, diced
- 1 onion, chopped

Directions:
⇒ Add all ingredients except quinoa into a cooking pot and stir well.
⇒ Cover and cook on medium heat for 1 hour.
⇒ After 1 hour cook on low for 40 minutes
⇒ Stir well and serve.

Nutrition Facts per Serving :
Calories: 197 kcals, **Carbohydrates**: 33g, **Protein:** 9g, **Fat:** 5g, **Sodium:** 849mg, **Potassium:** 733mg, **Phosphorus:** 235mg

Stuffed Bell Pepper

Vegetarian-friendly
Gluten- free
Preparation Time: 15 minutes
Cooking Time: 25 minutes
Servings: 2

Ingredients:
- 2 medium bell peppers, cut in half and deseeded
- 2 tablespoons olive oil
- ¼ cup broccoli florets
- ¼ cup cherry tomatoes
- 1 teaspoon dried sage
- 1 oz cheddar cheese, grated
- Black pepper, to taste

Directions:
⇒ Preheat the oven to 390 F.
In a bowl, whisk together eggs, milk, broccoli, cherry tomatoes, sage, pepper.
⇒ Add oil to the baking dish and spread well. Place bell pepper halves in the baking dish.
⇒ Pour egg mixture into the bell pepper halves. Sprinkle cheese on top of bell pepper.
⇒ Bake for 25 minutes.
⇒ Serve.

Nutrition Facts per Serving:
Calories: 173 kcals, **Carbohydrates**: 5g, **Protein:** 8g, **Fat:** 14g, **Sodium:** 113mg, **Potassium:** 229mg, **Phosphorus:** 140mg

Zucchini Eggplant with Cheese

Vegetarian-friendly
Preparation Time: 15 minutes
Cooking Time: 40 minutes
Servings: 3

Ingredients:
- 1 medium eggplant, sliced
- 1 tablespoon olive oil
- 1 cup cherry tomatoes, halved
- 4 garlic cloves, minced
- 4 tablespoons basil, chopped
- 3 medium zucchinis, sliced
- 3 oz cottage cheese,
- ½ teaspoon black pepper

Directions:
⇒ Preheat the oven to 350 F.
⇒ Spray baking dish with cooking spray.
⇒ In a large bowl add chopped cherry tomatoes, eggplant, zucchini, olive oil, garlic, cheese, basil, pepper, and stir well.
⇒ Transfer the eggplant mixture into the baking dish and place dish in the oven.
⇒ Bake for 35 minutes.
⇒ Serve and enjoy.

Nutrition Facts per Serving:
Calories: 11 kcals, **Carbohydrates**: 13g, **Protein:** 6g, **Fat:** 5g, **Sodium:** 93mg, **Potassium:** 711mg, **Phosphorus:** 125mg

Chapter 13. Desserts

Chocolate Beet Cake

Preparation Time: 60 minutes
Cooking Time: 45 minutes
Servings: 6

Ingredients:
- 2 cups grated beets
- ¼ cup sunflower oil
- 1 egg
- 4 oz. unsweetened chocolate
- 2 tsp. phosphorus-free baking powder
- 2 cups all-purpose flour
- 1 cup sugar

Directions:
⇒ Set your oven to 325°F. Grease two 8-inch cake pans.
⇒ Mix the baking powder, flour, and sugar together. Set aside.
⇒ Chop up the chocolate as finely as you can and melt using a double boiler. A microwave can also be used, but don't let it burn.
⇒ Allow it to cool, and then mix in the oil and eggs.
⇒ Mix all of the wet ingredients into the flour mixture and combine everything together until well mixed.
⇒ Fold the beets in and pour the batter into the cake pans.
⇒ Let them bake for 40 to 50 minutes. To know it's done, the toothpick should come out clean when inserted into the cake.
⇒ Remove from the oven and allow them to cool.
⇒ Once cool, invert over a plate to remove.
⇒ This is great when served with whipped cream and fresh berries. Enjoy!

Nutrition Facts per Serving:
Calories: 514 kcals, **Carbohydrates:** 75g, **Protein:** 9g, **Fat:** 20g, **Sodium:** 52mg, **Potassium:** 360mg, **Phosphorus:** 153mg

Strawberry Pie

Preparation Time: 15 minutes
Cooking Time: 3 hours 25 minutes
Servings: 6

Ingredients:
- 1 1/2 cups Graham cracker crumbs
- 5 tbsp. unsalted butter, at room temperature
- 2 tbsp. sugar

For the Pie:
- 1 ½ teaspoon gelatin powder
- 3 tablespoons cornstarch
- ¾ cup sugar
- 5 cups sliced strawberries, divided
- 1 cup water

Directions:
⇒ For the crust: heat your oven to 375°F. Grease a pie pan.
⇒ Combine the butter, crumbs, and sugar together, and then press them into your pie pan.
⇒ Bake the crust for 10 to 15 minutes, until lightly browned.
⇒ Take out of the oven and let it cool completely.

For the pie:
⇒ Crush up a cup of strawberries.
⇒ Using a small pot, combine the sugar, water, gelatin, and cornstarch.
⇒ Bring the mixture in the pot up to a boil, lower the heat, and simmer until it has thickened.
⇒ Add in the crushed strawberries in the pot and let it simmer for another 5 minutes until the sauce has thickened up again.
⇒ Set it off the heat and pour it into a bowl.
⇒ Cool until it comes to room temperature.
⇒ Blend the remaining berries with the sauce so that it is well distributed and pour into the pie crust and spread it out into an even layer.
⇒ Refrigerate the pie until cold. This will take about 3 hours. Serve and enjoy!

Nutrition Facts per Serving:
Calories: 247 kcals, **Carbohydrates:** 49g, **Protein:** 2g, **Fat:** 11g, **Sodium:** 61mg, **Potassium:** 210mg, **Phosphorus:** 34mg

Pumpkin Cheesecake

Vegetarian-friendly recipe
Preparation Time: 1 hour 10 minutes
Cooking Time: 20 minutes
Servings: 6

Ingredients:
- 1 egg white
- 1 wafer crumb, 9-inch pie crust
- ½ cup granulated sugar
- ½ teaspoon vanilla extract
- ½ small bowl liquid egg substitute
- 12 oz. cream cheese
- ½ cup pumpkin puree

Directions:
⇒ Brush pie crust with egg white and cook for 5 minutes in a preheated oven from 375°F from 375°F, now down to 350°F.
⇒ In a large cup, put together sugar, vanilla, and cream cheese, beating with a mixer until smooth.
⇒ Beat the egg substitute and add pumpkin puree with pie flavoring: blend everything until softened.
⇒ Put the pumpkin mixture in a pie shell and bake for 50 minutes to set the center.
⇒ Then let the pie cool down and then put it in the fridge. When you wish to, serve it in 8 slices, putting some topping on it.
⇒ Serve and enjoy!

Nutrition Facts per Serving:
Calories: 301 kcals, **Carbohydrates:** 22g, **Protein:** 8g, **Fat:** 21g, **Sodium:** 225mg, **Potassium:** 150mg, **Phosphorus:** 123mg

Small Chocolate Cakes

Preparation Time: 10 minutes
Cooking Time: 20 minutes
Servings: 6

Ingredients:
- 2 eggs, beaten
- 5 tablespoons butter
- 5 oz small squared dark chocolate
- 5 tablespoons cake flour
- non-stick cooking spray

Directions:
⇒ Preheat the oven to 350°F.
⇒ Melt butter and chocolate dark in small saucepan and let it cool for 5 minutes.
⇒ In a food processor beat the eggs for 3 minutes.
⇒ Add flour and blend. Pour chocolate and butter mixture in the food processor.
⇒ Put the mix in a mold and bake for 20 minutes.
⇒ Slip the cupcake out of the mold and put it on a dish, let it cool.
⇒ Serve and enjoy.

Nutrition Facts per Serving:
Calories: 321 kcals, **Carbohydrates:** 69g, **Protein:** 5g, **Fat:** 4g, **Sodium:** 627mg, **Potassium:** 128mg, **Phosphorus:** 275mg

Strawberry Whipped Cream Cake

Preparation Time: 20 minutes
Cooking Time: 0 minutes
Servings: 6
Preparation Time: 30 Minutes

Ingredients:
- 1 pint whipped cream
- 2 tablespoons gelatin
- ½ glass cold water
- 1 glass boiling water
- 3 tablespoons lemon juice
- 1 teaspoons sugar
- ¾ cup sliced strawberries
- 1 large angel food cake or light sponge cake

Directions:
⇒ Put the gelatin in cold water, then add hot water and blend. Add lemon juice, also add some sugar and go on blending.
⇒ Refrigerate and leave it there until you see it is starting to gel.
⇒ Whip half portion of cream and add it to the mixture along with strawberries, put wax paper in the bowl, and cut the cake into small pieces.
⇒ In between the pieces, add the whipped cream and put everything in the fridge for 10-12 hours.
⇒ When you take out the cake, add some whipped cream on top and decorate with some more fruit.
⇒ Serve and enjoy!

Nutrition Facts per Serving:
Calories: 462 kcals, **Carbohydrates:** 32g, **Protein:** 8g, **Fat:** 35g, **Sodium:** 381mg, **Potassium:** 172mg, **Phosphorus:** 213mg

Sweet Cracker Pie Crust

Diabetes-friendly recipe
Preparation Time: 15 minutes
Cooking Time: 20 minutes
Servings: 2

Ingredients:
- 1 bowl gelatin cracker crumbs
- 1/4 small cup sugar
- 3 teaspoons unsalted butter

Directions:
⇒ Preheat the oven to 375°F.
⇒ Mix sweet cracker crumbs, butter, and sugar.
⇒ Put in a baking tray and then in the oven.
⇒ Bake for 7 minutes.
⇒ Let the pie cool before adding any kind of filling.
⇒ Serve and enjoy.

Nutrition Facts per Serving:
Calories: 145 kcals, **Carbohydrates:** 25g, **Protein:** 1g, **Fat:** 6g, **Sodium:** 1mg, **Potassium:** 2mg, **Phosphorus:** 2mg

Apple Oatmeal Crunchy

Preparation Time: 10 minutes
Cooking Time: 20 minutes
Servings: 6

Ingredients:
- 5 green apples
- 1 bowl oatmeal
- A small cup brown sugar
- ½ cup flour
- 1 teaspoon cinnamon
- ½ cup butter

Directions:
⇒ Prepare apples by cutting them into tiny slices and preheat the oven at 350°F.
⇒ In a cup, mix oatmeal, flour, cinnamon, and brown sugar.
⇒ Put butter in the batter and place sliced apple in a baking pan (9" x 13").
⇒ Spread oatmeal mixture over the apples and bake for 35 minutes. Serve and enjoy!

Nutrition Facts per Serving:
Calories: 227 kcals, **Carbohydrates:** 55g, **Protein:** 2g, **Fat:** 1g, **Sodium:** 10mg, **Potassium:** 220mg, **Phosphorus:** 30mg

Berry Ice Cream

Preparation Time: 10 minutes
Cooking Time: 0 minutes
Servings: 6

Ingredients:
- 6 ice cream cones
- 1 cup whipped topping
- 1 cup fresh blueberries
- 4 oz. cream cheese
- 1/4 cup blueberry jam

Directions:
⇒ Put the cream cheese in a large cup and beat it with a mixer until it is fluffy.
⇒ Mix with fruit and jam and whipped topping.
⇒ Put the mixture on the small ice cream cones and refrigerate them in the freezer for 2 hours.
⇒ Serve and enjoy.

Nutrition Facts per Serving:
Calories: 177 kcals, **Carbohydrates:** 21g, **Protein:** 3g, **Fat:** 10g, **Sodium:** 91mg, **Potassium:** 72mg, **Phosphorus:** 43mg

Blueberry Peach Crisp

Preparation Time: 10 minutes
Cooking Time: 45 minutes
Servings: 6

Ingredients:
- 7 medium-sized fresh peaches
- 1 cup blueberries
- ¼ cup granulated sugar
- 1 tablespoon lemon juice
- ¾ cup all-purpose flour
- ¾ cup packed brown sugar
- ½ cup butter

Directions:
⇒ Preheat oven to 375°F
⇒ Pit and slice the peaches into ¾- inch slices
⇒ Use a cooking spray to spray a 12 x 9-inch baking dish, then place the peach slices and blueberries on top of the dish
⇒ Sprinkle over the fruit, sugar, and lemon juice
⇒ Use a small bowl to combine and mix the flour and brown sugar
⇒ Cut the butter into the flour mixture using two knives or pastry blender until it is crumbly. Sprinkle the crumbs on top of the fruit

⇒ Bake for about 45 minutes or until the fruit becomes soft and the crumbs are browned, then serve warm.

Nutrition Facts per Serving:
Calories: 353 kcals, **Carbohydrates:** 54g, **Protein:** 3g, **Fat:** 15g, **Sodium:** 9mg, **Potassium:** 261mg, **Phosphorus:** 45mg

Cherry Coffee Cake

Preparation Time: 10 minutes
Cooking Time: 40 minutes
Servings: 6

Ingredients:
- ½ cup unsalted butter
- 1 egg
- 1 cup granulated sugar
- 1 cup sour cream
- 1 teaspoon vanilla
- 1 cup all-purpose white flour
- 1 teaspoon baking powder
- 1 teaspoon baking soda
- 5 ounces cherry pie filling

Directions:
⇒ Preheat the oven to 350°F
⇒ Set out the butter at room temperature to soften
⇒ Use a bowl to cream the butter, eggs, sour cream, sugar, and vanilla
⇒ Combine and mix the flour, baking powder, and baking soda in a separate bowl
⇒ Add the dry ingredients from step 4 to the creamed butter mixture. Mix properly, then pour the batter onto a greased 9 x 13-inch baking pan
⇒ Evenly spread the cherry pie filling over the batter
⇒ Bake for about 40 minutes or until it is golden brown

Nutrition Facts per Serving:
Calories: 439 kcals, **Carbohydrates:** 58g, **Protein:** 4g, **Fat:** 22g, **Sodium:** 110mg, **Potassium:** 154mg, **Phosphorus:** 120mg

Fruity Peach Crisp Dump

Preparation Time: 10 minutes
Cooking Time: 30 minutes
Servings: 6

Ingredients:
- 10 ounces of sliced canned peaches
- Non-stick cooking spray
- 1 egg
- ½ cup all-purpose flour
- ½ cup butter, melted
- ½ cup skimmed milk
- ½ cup brown sugar
- ½ teaspoon baking soda

Directions:
⇒ Preheat oven to 350°F
⇒ Spray the cooking spray over a 9 x 13-inch cake pan
⇒ Dump two cans of undrained peaches onto the cake pan, spreading evenly
⇒ With a food processor blend egg, flour, butter, milk, sugar and baking soda for 1 minute.
⇒ Pour the batter on top of the fruit.
⇒ Bake for about 35 minutes.
⇒ Cut in slices and serve warm.

Nutrition Facts per Serving:
Calories: 286 kcals, **Carbohydrates:** 33g, **Protein:** 3g, **Fat:** 17g, **Sodium:** 30mg, **Potassium:** 146mg, **Phosphorus:** 73mg

Gingersnap Cookies

Preparation Time: 10 minutes
Cooking Time: 1 hour 10 minutes
Servings: 6

Ingredients:
- 2 cups all-purpose white flour
- 3 teaspoons baking soda
- 1 teaspoon ground ginger
- 1 teaspoon ground cinnamon
- 1 stick unsalted softened butter
- 1 cup granulated sugar
- 1 egg
- 2 tablespoons molasses

Directions:
- Sift together the flour, baking soda, ginger and cinnamon
- Cream the butter using a mixer until it becomes light and fluffy, add sugar gradually, then blend in the egg and molasses
- Pour in a little amount of the flour mixture at a time until a dough is formed
- Cover and store in the refrigerator for 1 hour or overnight
- Preheat oven to 350°F
- Form the dough into a heaped teaspoon ball size, and place 2-inch apart on top of a greased cookie sheet. Slightly flatten each ball.

- o Bake for about 8 to 10 minutes, then cool on a wire rack.
- o Serve and enjoy.

Nutrition Facts per Serving:
Calories: 450 kcals, **Carbohydrates:** 72g, **Protein:** 5g, **Fat:** 16g, **Sodium:** 18mg, **Potassium:** 316mg, **Phosphorus:** 170mg

Lemon Icebox Pie

Preparation Time: 4 hours 10 minutes
Cooking Time: 20 minutes
Servings: 6

Ingredients:
- o ½ cup water
- o 1 small packet Knox unflavored gelatin
- o 8 ounces light sour cream
- o 2½ cups fat-free Reddi-Wip dairy whipped topping
- o ¼ cup lemon juice
- o ⅓ cup granulated sugar
- o ¼ teaspoon lemon extract
- o 6 drops of yellow food coloring
- o 1 Graham (9-inch) cracker pie crust

Directions:
⇒ Dissolve the gelatin into ½ cup of boiling water, and allow it to stand for about five minutes.
⇒ Combine and mix the sour cream, 2 cups of whipped topping, lemon juice, sugar, lemon extract, and food coloring. Stir in the dissolved gelatin.
⇒ Pour the mixture into a pie shell, and store in the refrigerator for about 4 hours or until it is set.
⇒ Cut into slices, topping each with one tablespoon of the remaining whipped topping.

Nutrition Facts per Serving:
Calories: 308 kcals, **Carbohydrates:** 36g, **Protein:** 5g, **Fat:** 17g, **Sodium:** 169mg, **Potassium:** 160mg, **Phosphorus:** 83mg

Strawberry Pavlova

Preparation Time: 30 minutes
Cooking Time: 1 hour 15 minutes
Servings: 6

Ingredients:
- o 6 large egg white
- o 2 cups+ 2 tablespoons granulated sugar
- o 1½ teaspoons vinegar
- o 2½ teaspoons vanilla extract
- o 8 ounces of light whipping cream
- o 4 cups fresh sliced strawberries

Directions:
⇒ Preheat oven to 300°F.
⇒ Set out the egg white at room temperature; slice the strawberries and keep aside.
⇒ Beat the egg white with salt until soft peaks are formed. Add 2 cups of sugar, one tablespoon at a time, and beat properly after each addition. Fold in the vinegar gently, adding 1½ teaspoons of vanilla.
⇒ Use an 8-inch round and ungreased cookie sheet to smooth in the mixture.
⇒ Bake for about 45 minutes, then allow the shell to set for about 1 hour with the oven door closed. Remove from the oven, allowing it to cool completely.
⇒ Add sugar, whipping cream, and the remaining 1 teaspoon of vanilla into a bowl, whipping with a mixer until it becomes stiff. Place the whipped cream in the freezer for about 10–15 minutes.
⇒ Fill the top of the Pavlova shell from step 5 with the whipped topping and sliced berries.

Nutrition Facts per Serving:
Calories: 421 kcals, **Carbohydrates:** 76g, **Protein:** 5g, **Fat:** 12g, **Sodium:** 63mg, **Potassium:** 246mg, **Phosphorus:** 53mg

Snickerdoodles

Preparation Time: 15 minutes
Cooking Time: 10 minutes
Servings: 6

Ingredients:
- o 1 cup all-purpose white flour
- o 1 ½ cup sugar (divided use)
- o 1 egg
- o ¾ teaspoon cream tartar
- o 1 tablespoon unsalted butter
- o ½ teaspoon baking soda
- o 2 teaspoons vanilla
- o 1½ teaspoon ground cinnamon

Directions:
⇒ Preheat oven to 400°F.
⇒ Use a large bowl to combine and mix all the cookie ingredients, excluding the cinnamon and leaving out ¼ of the sugar.
⇒ Using a small bowl, stir in the remaining sugar and the cinnamon.
⇒ Form 1-inch of balls and roll into the sugar mixture.

⇒ Use an ungreased cookie sheet to place in the dough balls, 2-inch apart.
⇒ Bake for about 8 to 10 minutes or until it is browned.
⇒ Serve and enjoy.

Nutrition Facts per Serving:
Calories: 302 kcals, **Carbohydrates:** 50g, **Protein:** 3g, **Fat:** 3g, **Sodium:** 12mg, **Potassium:** 126mg, **Phosphorus:** 55mg

Bread Pudding

Preparation Time: 15 minutes
Cooking Time: 40 minutes
Servings: 6

Ingredients:
o   2 eggs
o   2 egg whites
o   1½ cups almond milk
o   2 tablespoons honey
o   1 teaspoon vanilla
o   2 tablespoons rum or 1 teaspoon rum extract
o   4 slices raisin bread

Directions:
⇒ Preheat oven to 325° F
⇒ Use a non-stick cooking spray to spray an 8-inch round baking dish
⇒ Beat the eggs and egg white in a large mixing bowl until it is foamy. Beat in the almond milk, vanilla, honey, and the rum or rum extract
⇒ Cut the bread into cubes, stir into the egg mixture then spread over the baking dish
⇒ Bake for about 35 to 40 minutes or until it comes out clean when a knife is inserted at the center
⇒ Spoon out warm pudding into dishes to serve.

Nutrition Facts per Serving:
Calories: 105 kcals, **Carbohydrates:** 16g, **Protein:** 4g, **Fat:** 2g, **Sodium:** 111mg, **Potassium:** 89mg, **Phosphorus:** 44mg

Frozen Fruit Delight

Preparation Time: 3 hours
Cooking Time: 0 minutes
Servings: 6

Ingredients:
o   ⅓ cup maraschino cherries
o   8 ounces pineapple, canned and crushed
o   8 ounces reduced-fat sour cream
o   1 tablespoon lemon juice
o   1 cup strawberries, sliced
o   ½ cup sugar
o   ⅛ teaspoon salt
o   3 cups dairy whipped topping

Directions:
⇒ Chop the cherries and drain the pineapple
⇒ Place all the ingredients into a medium-sized bowl except the whipped topping. Mix until well blended, then fold in the whipped topping.
⇒ Place the mixture into a freezable plastic container.
⇒ Freeze for about 3 hours.
⇒ Serve and enjoy

Nutrition Facts per Serving:
Calories: 256 kcals, **Carbohydrates:** 35g, **Protein:** 4g, **Fat:** 12g, **Sodium:** 78mg, **Potassium:** 213mg, **Phosphorus:** 36mg

Italian Tiramisu Cheesecake

Diabetes-friendly
Preparation Time: 45 minutes
Cooking Time: 0 minutes
Servings: 10

Ingredients:
o   6 egg whites, whipped
o   10 ounces mascarpone cheese
o   ½ cup sugar
o   1 teaspoon vanilla extract
o   4 ounces brewed espresso
o   1 tablespoon bitter cocoa powder

Directions:
⇒ Cut the pound cake into ten even slices, and set aside
⇒ Mix the cheese, vanilla, and sugar in a bowl until it is smooth. Add the whipped eggs.
⇒ Pour the espresso into a shallow dish
⇒ Dip the sides of 4 pieces of pound cake into the espresso, placing them in an 8-inch loaf pan. Break the pieces up, if required to coat the bottom of the pan
⇒ Gently spread ⅓ of the cream cheese mixture over the cake. Repeat procedure with the remaining slices of pound cake to make three layers.
⇒ Sprinkle cocoa powder on top.
⇒ Refrigerate for about 3 hours, then cut into pieces of 10 and serve

Nutrition Facts per Serving:
Calories: 174 kcals, **Carbohydrates:** 12g, **Protein:** 4g, **Fat:** 13g, **Sodium:** 53mg, **Potassium:** 105mg, **Phosphorus:** 24mg

Frozen Lemon Dessert

Preparation Time: 10 minutes
Cooking Time: 10 minutes
Servings: 2

Ingredients:
- 4 eggs, separated
- ¼ cup lemon juice
- 2/3 cup sugar
- 1 tablespoon lemon peel, grated
- 2 cups vanilla wafers, crushed
- 1 cup whipped cream

Directions:
⇒ Beat the egg yolks until they become very thick.
⇒ Slowly add sugar and beat each time you add.
⇒ Add the lemon peel and lemon juice, mix well.
⇒ Put the mixture in a double boiler and cook over boiling water, constantly stirring until the mixture gets thick.
⇒ Take off heat and keep aside to cool.
⇒ Beat the egg whites until stiff.
⇒ Pour the egg whites into the thick mixture once cooled. Add whipped cream and stir.
⇒ Spread one and a half crumbs of the vanilla wafer in the bottom of a baking dish or freezer tray.
⇒ Scoop the lemon mixture and spread over the crumbs.
⇒ Sprinkle the remaining vanilla wafer crumbs on the top.
⇒ Freeze for 5 hours until the mixture is firm.

Nutrition Facts per Serving:
Calories: 387 kcals, **Carbohydrates:** 44g, **Protein:** 6g, **Fat:** 22g, **Sodium:** 139mg, **Potassium:** 117mg, **Phosphorus:** 106mg

Chocolate Pie Shell

Preparation Time: 40 minutes
Cooking Time: 40 minutes
Servings: 6

Ingredients:
- 3 cups Cocoa Krispies, crushed
- 4 tablespoons butter
- Cooking spray

Directions:
⇒ Crush the cocoa Krispies, melt the butter and add both to a bowl and stir.
⇒ Spray a 9-inch pie pan with cooking spray, then press the mixture into the pie pan.
⇒ Place in the refrigerator to chill for a minimum of 30 minutes before filling.
⇒ You can add any filling of your choice

Nutrition Facts per Serving:
Calories: 78 kcals, **Carbohydrates:** 11g, **Protein:** 1g, **Fat:** 10g, **Sodium:** 48mg, **Potassium:** 23mg, **Phosphorus:** 12mg

Conclusion

Chronic kidney disease is a severe condition that affects millions of people worldwide. Kidneys filter excess water and waste from the blood, but when kidneys are damaged, they cannot perform this function effectively. This can lead toxins to build up in your body, causing various health problems.

One of the most effective ways to feel better with chronic kidney disease is diet. Following a renal diet can support kidney function and lower the risk of complications related to kidney disease. A renal diet typically involves reducing the intake of foods high in sodium and potassium and limiting the protein and phosphorus intake.

The kidney diet recipes in this book are specifically designed to help people with chronic kidney disease manage their condition. These recipes are low in protein, sodium, potassium, and phosphorus and high in fiber and other essential nutrients.

Adding these recipes to your diet allows you to enjoy a wide range of delicious, kidney-friendly meals that will help you maintain good health and improve kidney function.
I hope I have set you on the right path to selecting and preparing a delicious meal to help improve your kidneys' health. These Renal Diet recipes are perfect for sharing with the whole family.

Keep practicing and exploring new and exciting meals from this book. Mix and match the delicious recipes to create your favorite Renal Diet meal and get over 1,500 kidney-friendly days.
You can return to this guidebook any time you doubt or want to get back to valuable tips on living a healthier life with damaged renal functions and chronic kidney disease. The state of your renal function defines how well your body is functioning; however, as explained in the book, your health should see crucial improvements with the change in your diet.
Make sure always to check your labels when shopping for groceries and ensure that the meals you are preparing are ready by the low-potassium and low-sodium diets for best results.
Remember, making healthy choices is essential for everyone but especially important for people with chronic kidney disease. You can improve your functioning and live a happier and more fulfilling life. Keep practicing, discover new and exciting dishes from this book, and care for your health today.

Made in the USA
Middletown, DE
14 June 2023

32631805R00053